PAWS
noses & people

A history of Dogs for the Disabled and the
development of assistance dogs in the UK

DICK LANE

PAWS
noses & people

A history of Dogs for the Disabled and the
development of assistance dogs in the UK

DICK LANE

MEREO
Cirencester

Mereo Books

1A The Wool Market Dyer Street Cirencester Gloucestershire GL7 2PR
An imprint of Memoirs Publishing www.mereobooks.com

PAWS, noses and people: 978-1-86151-487-5

First published in Great Britain in 2015
by Mereo Books, an imprint of Memoirs Publishing

The address for Memoirs Publishing Group Limited can be found at
www.memoirspublishing.com

The Memoirs Publishing Group Ltd Reg. No. 7834348

The Memoirs Publishing Group supports both The Forest Stewardship Council® (FSC®)
and the PEFC® leading international forest-certification organisations. Our books
carrying both the FSC label and the PEFC® and are printed on FSC®-certified paper.
FSC® is the only forest-certification scheme supported by the leading environmental
organisations including Greenpeace. Our paper procurement policy can be found at
www.memoirspublishing.com/environment

Typeset in 9/15pt Franklin Gothic by Wiltshire Associates Publisher Services Ltd. Printed
and bound in Great Britain by Printondemand-Worldwide, Peterborough PE2 6XD

Contents

Acknowledgments

I would like to thank Bonita Bergin, Rosemary Smith, George Newns, Bruce Jones, Sheila Sills, Anne Greenwood, Wendy Morrell, Jenny Donnely-Thompson, Wendy Robinson, Angela Heeley. Also all those who gave their time for interviews and dog reports to help in the book's production: M1 Photofile; Banbury Guardian; Colan (all for photos). Any errors of fact or opinion are mine and in no way the fault of the many contributors who in various ways have made this book possible.

Dick Lane MSc FRCVS
Vice President, Dogs for the Disabled
York, England

Introduction

It is now over 25 years since the first assistance dog was trained in Great Britain, for a lady with the disability of being a double amputee. Based on my personal memories, interviews with people who have used dogs and from the detailed minutes kept by the charity Dogs for the Disabled which is at the heart of this book, the story evolves of how dogs have been used in many helping ways, far beyond the hopes of Frances Hay, who founded the first charity in England to train such a specialist dog.

On a quiet afternoon in 1991, the phone rang in my veterinary surgery at Leamington Spa; a not unexpected experience, as afternoon surgery had just finished and it was time to think of routine calls that might be waiting. But this call was different: in effect, would I go out to the nearby town of Kenilworth and collect a body off the railway line.

The veterinary student who was attending the veterinary practice for practical instruction responded with a 'why us?', a response to the feeling that was creeping into the minds of the more science-based veterinary undergraduates.

The art and science, coupled with public service ethos, was slowly dwindling in veterinary practice as subjects such as business skills and technical competence took a greater part in student training. I had to point out that this call was to a dog called Amie which had belonged to the recently-deceased Frances Hay, who had founded an organisation called 'Dogs for the Disabled' some years previously. Her dogs had been taken to Crackley Woods to exercise by Frances' daughter, a young person well used to dog handling. Unfortunately

Amie, a lively Golden Retriever, had decided to run off, and met a quick end under the wheels of a passing goods train.

The student and I arrived at Frances' house, and after being instructed by Frances' father as to where the dog was last seen, I set off into the woods, following well-used paths. The student followed behind was carrying the necessary black plastic bag, and ignoring railway safety procedures that required vets (and all others) to wear a high-visibility jacket.

We approached the railway track, and there between the rails were the remains of Amie. Anyone who has dealt with animals that get under trains knows that the flailing action of wheels passing over removes loose appendages, but the collar still on the dog was confirmation that this indeed was the iconic Amie.

Such self-destruction seems to have accompanied much of Frances' life. She was an only child, her parents travelling abroad with the British Diplomatic Service postings in the post-war period. When she was a young teenager in Singapore, a lump on the leg had been diagnosed as bone cancer, and her father moved to Australia; later the leg had to be cut off above the knee. She did not allow the amputation to restrict her enthusiasm for life, although in her latter years she may have realised she had less time left than others to make a mark on the world.

I first met Frances Hay in 1986, when she was living in an end-of-terrace Edwardian house with two dogs and a teenage daughter. I had just returned from the Delta Conference in Boston and had done some work with the Matron of a geriatric hospital at Whitnash near Warwick, involving animal therapies. Frances' family were involved and her father recognised the contribution made by his granddaughter at a time she was coping with school, exams and other difficulties: 'She was of course quite young at the time but she was very active in the development of the charity, being involved in filing, retrieving, dog walking, answering the phone, attending meetings at which Fran made speeches and probably a host of other things only she would know about.'

Frances once rode through Coventry on a horse, partially undressed as Lady Godiva! As a publicity stunt it made little impact on the finances of Dogs for the Disabled, but as a means of satisfying Frances' ego it was a brave act. Touring local pubs in and around Kenilworth with one of her friends, using collecting tins to raise funds, was another social activity she used to get herself known.

Frances' idea of forming a support dog organisation was probably influenced by the presence of the Guide Dogs for the Blind Association's original training centre in Leamington Spa. It was at Kenilworth that Frances realised that Kim, her first rescue dog, was helping her to balance as she walked with a stiff lead. The name 'Dogs for the Disabled' came to her mind as an attempt to promote the idea that dogs could give assistance to other people than the blind, people who also had special needs.

She set up an office in the basement of her own house and attracted two part-time workers for secretarial and dog-walking duties. The name stuck, and it was used when she was able to have a charity registered for this purpose. Despite murmurings of political correctness and the abolishment of the word 'handicapped', the successful charity she founded still uses the same title. The defence had always been that a person with a major disability had decided the title was appropriate, so it should remain in her memory.

The organisation Assistance Dogs (UK) includes the dog charities The Guide Dogs for the Blind Association and Hearing Dogs for Deaf Persons, but their histories have been written about elsewhere and they are only mentioned in this account when they are involved in the newer groups. Leading characters' names are written in full, but to provide a level of anonymity first names only have been used for many of the stories included in the book.

Chapter 1

From the first assistance dogs to a worldwide canine helper movement

It is only comparatively recently that the term 'assistance dog' has become recognised as one used for the group of various breeds trained to help humans for a specific purpose. In the 1930s attention was focused on the development of the use of dogs to help blind people, and the 'guide dog' term then became firmly established in the United Kingdom. The term 'Seeing Eye Dog' was used in North America, but not in Europe, where 'guide dog' was adopted by many countries.

In 1977, Dogs for the Deaf was founded in the USA by an animal trainer Roy Kabat. The dogs trained with persons became known as 'hearing dogs', a title that did not explain what they did to help people. More recently dogs are being trained and used to improve the quality of life for a wider variety of people with disabilities.

Still known as 'service dogs' in the USA, dogs for disability help have been trained and used in many countries of the world, and the number of such dogs and the uses they are put to continue to increase. 'Assistance dogs for mobility' was a title attributed to Bonita

Bergin in the USA to distinguish trained dogs from service dogs which were trained by the military there.

The casualties in wars have often led to the need for advances in human treatments, as in surgical and medical nursing. Blood and fluid transfusions, portable X-rays and immediate casualty care were all developed as military medicine. Chemotherapeutics originated from nerve gas agents used in warfare, while many of the earliest drugs used in cancer treatment were derived from such drugs, which are toxic to all cells. The mental injuries of battle fatigue and PTSD (known then as shell shock) received less attention, and psychiatric support was slower to develop to help such traumatised people.

Towards the end of the First World War in 1918, a German hospital doctor in Berlin recognised that his own dog was helping a blinded soldier to walk round the paths of the hospital gardens. In later wars spinal injuries and amputations, of military personnel, led to a need for dogs that could offer support and assistance to people. The Vietnam War of 1975 was associated with many battlefield injuries which resulted in the paralysis of fit young men, often known as 'vets', who needed mobility assistance and other aids for living.

The US military appointed Major Lynn Anderson of the Veterinary Corps to be the first consultant on the Human-Animal Bond (HAB) with an animal visitation programme at the medical facility in Washington of the United States Soldiers' and Airmen's Home. Since the recent conflicts in Iraq and Afghanistan began, the number of service people losing upper and lower limbs from explosive devices has brought greater public awareness of these severe disabilities, which with good support can return the injured to a near normal lifestyle. Advances such as bionic hands which give the patient the 'human touch' are just one development that can give these casualties, often quite young people, the opportunity to return to some form of active life.

The medical care of battlefield injuries with rapid evacuation to fully-equipped hospitals has markedly reduced death rates, but legs and arms may be lost, as amputations for survival may be the only course for surgeons to follow.

The assistance dogs could give was first recognised after the First World War, when there were massive casualties and ex-servicemen were sent home with severe physical and mental disabilities. Blindness from poisonous gases and explosives was one of many injuries that resulted from the conflict.

The story has been told elsewhere of how Dorothy Eustis in Switzerland started a school for guide dogs for the blind in the 1920s and how her dog trainers next came to the UK and the USA to set up the first of many guide dog training schools from the 1930s onwards. Influenced by the surge of blindness injuries during the Second World War, there was a further expansion, with many new dog schools opening in the USA.

In Britain one organisation, the Guide Dogs for the Blind Association, developed in the inter-war period. It remained the sole provider of dogs for the thousands of visually-impaired people in England, Wales, Scotland and Northern Ireland for over 75 years.

Assistance dogs trained to help deaf people was the next development, bringing in the idea of dogs that provided a service. In the USA, Agnes McGrath was credited as the first person to train dogs to assist people who were deaf or hard of hearing. The first such training school started in Minnesota and within its first year of operation, the school was taken over by the American Humane Association in Colorado. Although this arrangement did not survive for long, it influenced all other hearing dog schools to source their dogs from animal shelters and rescue kennels. They were not purpose bred for their work; unlike the larger breeds selected for work as guide dogs and later on dogs for wheelchair users, hearing dogs could be

3

any shape or size. Very often the smaller breeds were most suited to life with elderly hearing impaired persons who might not have gardens or recreation areas to provide for necessary exercise for larger or more active breeds.

The British Hearing Dogs for the Deaf, as it was first called, was based just outside London on the edge of the Chilterns, started in 1982 with a launch at a dog show in London. It became a registered charity in 1986 and slowly progressed in helping with deafness with the name Hearing Dogs for the Deaf, only recently renamed to become Hearing Dogs for Deaf Persons. At that time there were no other assistance dog organisations in England other than these two, which had restricted themselves to providing dogs for the visually impaired and deaf.

Meanwhile developments were taking place in the late twentieth century in North America which would influence the whole global scene of working assistance dogs.

Bonita (Bonnie) Bergin in the USA will always be associated with the idea of the next development stage of assistance, especially in the use of dogs for those in wheelchairs or having similar mobility problems. In 1975 the idea of dogs helping people with physical disabilities came to her whilst she was studying about disabilities as part of a Masters degree. She was a teacher and she wanted to help others. A 'mainstreaming law' had been passed in the USA that allowed access by individuals with disabilities to education, with entry into regular classrooms.

Bonita's research into dog personalities helped her in providing a basis for finding the right temperaments of animals; an objective in the concept of the service dog which was able to assist people with mobility limitations. She started the organisation Canine Companions for Independence (CCI) in Santa Rosa, California, to train and provide dogs. As time went on she expanded CCI to set up centres in New York, Ohio, Florida, and southern California.

4

In an account of her first 30 years developing the first non-profit organisation to train and place service dogs, Bonita Bergin recalls how she was inspired after working in Asia where animals such as small equids (ponies and donkeys) were being used by disabled persons to help them move round and to carry their possessions. When working in Turkey she recalled seeing a tetraplegic man propelling himself along by his elbows, his body dragging along behind; elsewhere limbless people sat on low wooden trolleys to provide them with limited mobility in the streets. Where wheelchairs were unavailable or even unknown such improvisation allows for a little freedom rather than total dependency or worse. In her own words:

'My thoughts were focused on the myriad of people with disabilities who couldn't do what I could do physically. I remembered people with disabilities using donkeys and burros to carry their pots and pans or other wares to street corners where they would sit down and sell them — functioning as part of the economic fabric of that country'.

One cannot consider the development of assistance dogs without describing another American pioneer, Kerry Knaus, whom I met in 1986 at a conference in Boston, USA. As a 19-year-old girl with a form of muscular dystrophy, Kerry had been dependent on her wheelchair for all physical movement, but she became involved in the work of the Community Resource Programme for Independence in Santa Rosa, California. As Bonita Bergin told me later, she had contacted the community organisation to ask if there was a person there who would be suitable for a project training a dog to help with disability. Kerry, who was working in an agency, was the one who immediately took up this challenge.

In one of those fortunate encounters during my life, I had arrived a day early in Boston and was curious when I saw in an upstairs corridor that was otherwise empty apart from a black Labrador beside a person in a wheelchair. It was later said to me that Kerry had a zest for living. Exploring and risk-taking were part of her mental outlook, and this was how I found her waiting when attending the Delta Conference.

The elderly-looking dog that accompanied her whilst in her wheelchair did enough to prompt my curiosity and I crossed the dark, empty passageway to greet the dog, introducing myself to Kerry. She told me she had had Abdul, a cross-bred Labrador and Golden Retriever puppy, since he was nine weeks old. Bred by Bonita Bergin, he had been trained to help her, and was her best friend.

Bonita later told me her first idea was that the puppy could be house trained and socialised by Kerry, before being old enough to commence his real training. Bonita wrote:

'Predictably, after a short stay in the home, the puppy had to be returned to Bonita as unmanageable. It was not Kerry's failure but the paid carer provided to help Kerry, who was not prepared to do the necessary mopping up of a puppy inside the house. Dramatically, the puppy had to be collected in the middle of the night to prevent a 'walk out' by the Government-paid care assistant who threatened to leave 'or else'. Subsequently there were training sessions provided twice a week by Bonita for Abdul and his intended new owner. In the summer, Kerry decided to take Abdul with her on vacation to her mother's home, where family members would be supportive and attend to Abdul's needs. After this bonding experience it became clear to Bonita that the two had developed such a strong association that it was not necessary for Abdul to be returned to her and the further training would continue in Kerry's home.

'Two other experienced dog trainers undertook this next stage and tasks such as retrieval, as well as walking and sitting to voice commands, developed quickly. Kerry found Dr Bonita Bergin, from her first experience of providing an assistance dog for a person in a wheelchair, had developed a new movement to use dogs. Kerry had identified tasks in which a dog could be of the greatest benefit to her. Many of these still form the basis of training a dog for specific needs of people: Bonita was able to ask Kerry about what her requirements were and what she could use a service dog for and her answers were precise and clear. What she needed was to have her dog pick up things that she dropped and that, she said, happened frequently, because her dexterity was so limited that she would readily drop a pen or pencil, or whatever item she was holding. She needed the item brought to her in such a way that she could slowly and carefully grasp it, because she didn't have the ability or the strength to grab for it or to hold it if it were the least bit heavy.

'Tasks as varied as picking up these dropped items to helping her go to the toilet were evaluated, as she thought a dog would help her. Specifically Kerry needed to have the lights turned on in the evenings when it became dark. If her attendant went out shopping in the day she might not return until after dark. She said that if she forgot to ask her attendant to turn them on for her she would then have to sit in the dark awaiting the carer's return. She needed help to have the remote control brought to her so the television could be turned on when she became bored from reading mid-afternoon and wanted a different form of entertainment.

'She needed a way to open doors, because she couldn't reach out and open them for herself. She would find herself feeling confined and want to have an alternative to her enclosed home environment, so she needed to be able to get outside in case of a fire or some other emergency. This is not an uncommon fear of persons suffering with various forms of disability, that escape from a threatening situation would be difficult or impossible. What Kerry needed in general was to be able to ask her dog to do things for her, so that she didn't constantly disturb the people around her with her small and seemingly petty needs.'

Bonita developed for her the 'visit' command, which had Abdul resting his chin on Kerry's lap and holding it still, so that Kerry could then take a retrieved item from his mouth, using her lap to help balance the item. This command also allowed her to stroke Abdul's face, virtually the only area of his body she could touch. One day, by using automatic controls to drive a van, she hoped to get more freedom and mobility. As an opportunity for independence, some of the capabilities that her physical limitations previously had made impossible for her were now within her horizon as she realised the potential of an assistance dog. She wanted to have her dog go with her wherever she went, to position himself to meet her needs, and for Abdul to lie down out of the way when she went into restaurants or to school so that other people were not stepping on him. Access issues would later be another problem to overcome.

At this pioneering stage, Kerry needed a dog who would accompany her anywhere. As an unobtrusive helpmate, a dog that would not cause difficulties would not be aggressive to friends and family, nor to people or other dogs walking on the street. Her dog should stay by her side and look for opportunities to help as she confronted each obstacle or difficulty in her life. She was fortunate in having Abdul, a dog who would gently lay his body across her lap so that she could warm her hands against his body. She said she required him to help nudge her head back up on her shoulders when it fell, since without sufficient muscle strength or movement, Kerry literally could not raise her head back up if it fell forward. She had so little circulation that even the tiniest of cold spells would cause her hands to freeze up, and what limited movement she had would be lost but for her dog's body heat; here too Abdul could help. It was not long before Abdul would bring her a cover to pull across her lap or take it away later, even being able to tug open a drawer, or to shut a room door was a godsend. In later years assistance dogs could be trained to help a client with dressing and undressing, removing sleeved garments from the shoulders or pulling off long socks.

Psychologically Kerry needed to have Abdul to be on view in public, to bring her presence to the attention of other people so that she would no longer be passed by, invisible in society. The social benefit of an assistance dog later could be proved, but it allowed Kerry to become a memorable and vibrant person, as I found her in the corridors of the Boston hotel where we first met and talked. She could now talk to people other than the rather limited group of those she had previously known in her church, in her family, or among her small circle of friends.

By appearing in public, she needed to show that a dog could do all these tasks, and do them without compromising its welfare. All dogs have willingness and a desire to please that could be harnessed to improve the quality of life of a person with physical disabilities. Abdul had made life worthwhile and pleasurable for her, in spite of physical limitations. It had been a bold move by Bonita Bergin and she was fortunate in her choice of Kerry with Abdul for this new venture. It was a tall order, but Abdul was the right dog to be able to comply with all these requirements.

This 'wants' list described by Kerry is not beyond the capability of the present-day assistance dog, but at that time it seemed she needed a dog to be more than just a robot that would follow all the commands and do all these duties. She needed him to be her best friend, her confidant and her partner in life.

Abdul was also the catalyst that led me to speak to Kerry first whilst waiting about in the corridor for my son, who was also at the conference. This meeting with Kerry later led me to seek out someone who had the idea of training such dogs in my own country. I was intrigued by the dog and the girl, articulate and willing to talk. I had told her about England and compared my experiences of working with

9

English guide dogs for 25 years with her use of a dog to help with another form of disability that differed from being visually 'handicapped'.

Later some additional tasks were described to me that could be developed by the user of an assistance dog using verbal praise and the occasional food reward. Kerry used a form of saddlebag, a cloth purse that an attendant of hers had made and fastened over Abdul's back like a pannier. It became apparent that one of Abdul's significant roles would be to carry items for Kerry. This became possible since he placed his front feet onto her feet on the wheelchair foot pedals, a position which placed his trunk in line with her lap so her hands could reach into the backpack and actually extract items that she normally would not have had the ability to reach or carry. Such a weight-carrying saddle was discouraged in the assistance dog movements. It led in later years to disrepute when a dog in one European country where a conference was in progress was seen out in the street carrying books in its back pack, at the same time limping from hip dysplasia.

Bonita wrote: 'Abdul, I have come to appreciate, was a dog and all that a dog can be. A wonderful dog who changed the world, who changed her life and in many ways showed the way into the future for assistance dogs. Thanks to Kerry's insight, perseverance and commitment, and Abdul's dedication to her, my dream of a service dog became a reality'.

After I met Kerry and Abdul on the day before the Delta Society International Conference started, she made an impression on other delegates coming to Boston in 1986, since she was one of the conference speakers who talked about the difference Abdul had made to her life. The thousand Delta Society delegates came mainly from North America, while there were other interested persons from overseas there as well, who had come to hear and participate in the Delta meeting. Bruce Fogle, James Serpell and Andrew Edney were other British speakers with me at the conference, all of whom have continued in various aspects of dog assistance activities.

On the final day all the British delegates were brought together for a group photo; many I did not realise had been there, as the gathering was so large. At the final meeting, a question was asked by an English person who I was later told was Anne Conway. She obviously had some knowledge about dog training and had been attending some of the talks. She was accompanied by veterinary surgeon Elizabeth Ormerod, who I met in a Boston breakfast bar, but over a coffee our interests seemed to differ once we got on to the subject of 'nurture'.

When I got back to England I wanted to find out why such activities and training for wheelchair users were not available in my own country. Then before the end of the same year I first heard about Frances Hay's work, already started in England. A local newspaper reported her attending an open day and fete at an NHS geriatric hospital in Leamington Spa in Warwickshire. I read that at Heathcote Hospital, Frances and the Hospital Matron, Mary Curran, were putting ideas together about using animals to help people into more stimulating activities.

I already knew Mrs Curran as a client. Years earlier she had initiated an early form of AAI (animal-assisted intervention), where donkeys were brought into the wards, dogs slept in the wards and young cats were allowed to jump onto the elderly patients' beds. There were six donkeys stabled outside, provided by the Donkey Trust. One pulled a cart used for patients to get fresh air and stimulation from being outside the wards. Others were led through the wards for patients to feel and touch. The dogs slept in the wards: Claire was a white collie, Cliff was a Golden Retriever obtained from the GDBA, there was a terrier, Sheba, and another white terrier, Judy. The cat population was two adults and two kittens; the latter were very popular for the very elderly to hold whilst lying in bed. There were also budgies and fish in tanks.

The first animals had been brought into the hospital in 1984. The average age of patients at Heathcote was 86, ranging from the youngest at 64 to the oldest at 104. I was there when the TV cameras of a national broadcaster came to see this phenomenon. The medical profession was generally opposed to animals coming into 'clean' hospital wards.

Mary Curran was eventually moved away to become an NHS nursing homes inspector and Heathcote patients were dispersed and the hospital buildings used for short-stay rehabilitation patients. It was a good example of AAI, and fortunately all the animals were taken into private homes by nurses and care workers.

Frances was not able to start her dog charity until 1988, and the struggle to get recognition and further the application of assistance dogs will be described in the next chapter with the many more developments that were to follow.

Four years after the Delta Conference meeting, Bonnie Bergin came to visit England and gave more help in developing the wider use of assistance dogs. In 1992 she was able to visit the Guide Dogs for the Blind Association's centre at Tollgate House to talk about her experiences when developing Canine Companions for Independence as a charity in the USA. The visit followed after the GDBA had showed an interest in service dog training and they financially supported a 'Bonita Bergin Service Dogs Seminar' in the States, by sending two employees, Helen McCain and Paul Master, to learn and contribute. Bonita was next invited to visit the GDBA when she was next in England for a conference. She came to Leamington Spa for her visit to the guide dog centre, and on her first to Warwickshire she described her methods and how she started her successful organisation. Her account was listened to closely and gave confidence to Dogs for the Disabled's Trustees, staff and other supporters there, who were just getting to a stage where the charity needed to grow.

From the very first, when training people and dogs at Santa Rosa with the charity Canine Companions for Independence, Bonita had experienced the difficulties of matching people to dogs to form lifelong partnerships. At first she used rescue or 'shelter' dogs and was putting them out with puppy socialisers, who had limited experience of training dogs from uncertain backgrounds. It caused so many problems that it led to the idea that it would be better to train puppies from a known background. The selection of puppies that could learn quickly, be energetic and responsive to humans would allow training to commence at eight weeks old rather than several months old.

Gradually Bonita realised that the key to improving the success rate for service dog training was to breed and raise her own puppies. Abdul, the first dog, had been bred following an accidental mating of her own Golden Retriever bitch with a neighbour's Labrador, a cross or hybrid which that the British guide dog school had already found produced trainable dogs with a better success rate than when either pure bred dog was used. At that time there was opposition amongst pedigree breeders to any puppies that did not have a 'pure line', and it was even held that subsequent litters bred by two of the same breed might produce 'tainted' puppies. Canine Companions found that breeding from healthy, low aroused Golden Retrievers and Labrador Retrievers was far from simple, but with experience matters improved.

Her first idea, of having potential clients rear and train puppies to provide a strong early bond between user and dog, proved impractical. The system was used years later for assistance dogs in Sweden in a 'self-training' process, using families with dog experience to take puppies into their own homes, in a process known as 'puppy walking,' from the way that fox hunting hounds were put out on farms, as 'walks'. The idea developed of using puppy socialisers who could provide the domestic background but also use their skills in providing early training for the future assistance dog. Known in the USA as 'volunteer puppy raisers', the arrangement allowed for a control of the puppies' environment and early learning at the critical stages of the pup's development.

Bonita continued her work in the United States over the next few decades, helping others with specifically-trained assistance dogs. She now runs the Bergin University of Canine Studies, the world's first accredited university in dog studies, involved in human and animal training in California. Her ideas on early socialisation and training puppies became widely accepted. As has been proved in subsequent years, nearly all Assistance Dogs International (ADI) instructors accept that the three or four-week-old puppy is capable of learning and benefit from handling away from the mother; they can develop attention to cues and wait until a treat is provided. USA Canine Companions trainers say that with puppies using their methods, it enables a trainer to fully train a puppy to respond to 90 service dog commands by about six months of age. The next twelve months of their development methods were spent with puppy handlers who fulfilled the need for the dog to have a wide range of public exposures and general socialisation. The puppy handlers then return the dog to kennels at 16 to 18 months for 'refresher' training, and then the placement with the client could begin.

In the post-World War II decades, the needs of the less able were recognised through the growing National Health Service providing disability facilities in the United Kingdom, but for some there was little encouragement for disabled persons to get into the workplace or become independent. Rarely were there special provisions for wheelchair users. Barriers to access in the form of high steps, lifts too narrow to take a person in a wheelchair and a lack of accessible public transport all tended to keep those in wheelchairs at home, perhaps relying on the occasional 'pusher' to give them an outing in the local park.

The scene has been slow to change during the last 50 years. Ludwig Guttmann, a refugee doctor from Breslau, had come to England in 1938, and he was asked by the wartime government to set up a spinal injuries unit at Stoke Mandeville Hospital near Aylesbury in 1944, to help injured ex-servicemen and others. The death rate of those with such injuries was 80% within the first year, while for the remainder the quality of their future life was poor. Guttmann set out to change this by encouraging activity supported by treatment; he started a small archery competition at the hospital in 1948, involving 16 paralysed British war veterans. This movement to encourage those with spinal injuries spread to other sports and led to the first 'Paralympics' in 1960. In Rome 400 wheelchair athletes paraded through the Olympic stadium for their own games competition, following the successful International Olympics held earlier that year.

The publicity following this athletic competition movement led to the need for more disability aids to be provided, better access for people with disabilities and a need for greater mobility. It took more than twenty years to grow, but eventually it would facilitate the 'Dogs for the Disabled' idea of Frances Hay in 1988, after she first used her own dog to give her greater mobility. This was some years after dogs were walking besides wheelchairs in the USA, but no attention had been given to using dogs in England for the purpose of doing anything more than providing companionship.

Chapter 2

Frances Hay's idea for a new dog charity

Frances Hay was the inspirational person whose vision led to the founding of the British assistance dog charity 'Dogs for the Disabled'. When she started the charity she fulfilled her wish to help others, held ever since she had had her left leg amputated and then had to depend on others as a schoolgirl at the age of 15. When bone cancer of her tibia was diagnosed, she had been given only two years to live, but she survived the next 25 years until her early death at the age of forty.

During her lifetime she made a considerable impact on the needs of many persons with disabilities. Fran, as she called herself, had developed a variety of interests during her life, but it was only quite late in her thirties that she conceived the idea of using a dog to help her with her own balance and mobility.

After living in London, a marriage in 1975 and then divorce brought her to live in Kenilworth, Warwickshire, with her dog Kim. Her choice of this small town close to Coventry was fortunate, since she was undoubtedly influenced by seeing in the locality the successful training programme of the Guide Dogs for the Blind Association (GDBA), based in nearby Leamington Spa. Dog trainers regularly walked their dogs on the streets of Leamington.

In the 1960s the GDBA were successfully raising money for their dog charity and had their own local support group nearby. The GDBA branch based in Leamington was a support group and raised money in regular street collections, and they ran a profitable summer fete each year at their training centre, Edmonscote Manor. The GDBA branch was led by Muriel Evans, whose own father had been using a guide dog trained to assist his mobility whilst blind; there was a lot of local support for dog training and it was a well-run charity.

It is unlikely that Muriel ever met Frances Hay; there was a strong loyalty in the area to all things relating to dogs for the blind, since it was the leading and predominating charity in the area, and this held back early attempts at seeking supporters or when collecting money for Dogs for the Disabled. After returning from the 1986 Boston Delta Conference, I read in the local newspaper about Frances attending the Heathcote Hospital open day and I contacted her by phone. I was surprised to find that there was a person using a 'support' dog in my own veterinary practice locality. My first letter to Frances was on November 18th 1986, written in reply to a letter she had sent to me two days earlier.

Letter from Frances dated 16th November 1986 when she sent cuttings from papers to explain what she was trying to do: 'Your views and your comments, along with any help that you might be able to give me will obviously be more than welcome. I look forward to hearing from you in the near future'.

Frances attached two copy letters from the Spastic Society and from Pedigree Petfoods, both of which showed their interest in Frances' ideas for using dogs. My reply to Frances was guarded: 'You have my moral support, but being involved in running the veterinary practice with other outside commitments as well, I am reluctant to take

17

up a new venture that involves more meetings, telephone calls at busy times or other calls on my limited free time. Please keep me informed and I would be willing to help in a small way: I would not wish to be Chairman of even a local group, since I know some of the problems that that can lead to with dissent amongst committee members!'

I was actively involved in the GDBA local branch and had also had the recent experience of setting up a local branch of the Cats Protection League (CPL) in Kenilworth. As the only man on the committee set up by Mary Caswell, the calls for help had intruded into my private life with factional disputes between the other committee members. After less than two years as the CPL Chairman, I had said either the secretary must go or I must go, so I chose to be the one to depart. I think this was why I was reluctant to engage in another new charity being set up.

In February 1987, a few friends of Frances had formed a support group for her embryo charity, which was based at Frances' own house in Kenilworth. It was a daunting task to set up a charity in a locality, as the area was very much focused on raising money for 'guide dogs'.

On February 27th 1987, Anne Conway wrote a letter to Frances which throws further light on how the two were diverging:

'Dear Frances, I have now received a letter from James Serpell. He says that the SCAS committee was somewhat divided over much they should be involved with our scheme, and cannot fund the project as SCAS has barely enough money for itself. Also he is too busy to give the project much more of his time, but Stuart Hutton had kindly agreed to take over. He feels as Stuart is a social worker he is better qualified – which could be right. James has asked me to inform him of the time and place of our meeting – but he says he is too busy to attend. As you will be aware from Stuart's letter, we ran into each other (sic) at Crufts and I had a long and interesting talk with him. He is is very interested in the scheme but he too has limited time. However I think he is willing to be involved at least in the early stages. He is an excellent treasurer for SCAS so perhaps he will also lend us a hand with the books?

'Elizabeth Ormerod, a veterinary surgeon from Lancashire I met at the Boston Conference last August, is also very keen on the scheme. She is very enthusiastic person and would be a great asset – and is able to inspire fundraisers in her area, also Lesley Scott Ordish, founder of PRO Dogs National charity, who is also responsible for creating the PAT dog programme, just might be interested in helping us to get started. She has lots of expertise on starting off charities as she is also the founder of HDFD.

'How we decide the date and the venue for the meeting. I wonder if you have heard from Alastair Mews and if we can get a room at the RSPCA in London. I am free any Monday or Tuesday in March and April, except 7 April. I look forward to hearing from you soon. Regards, (signed) Anne. PS: The problem of a suitable venue is solved (dated 22.2.87) I spoke to Heather Payne today who it is proposed should attend our meeting wearing her Pedigree Petfoods hat and she has said we could have a room at Gwynne Hart where she works in London. Heather has been involved in GDFD and was also at the Boston Conference and has therefore seen service/assistance dogs in action. Linda Hines, executive officer of the Delta Society (large American sister organisation of SCAS) will be in London in March and Heather thinks it could be a good idea to see if she can attend the meeting. Delta is very go-ahead and maybe it would act as an example to SCAS.'

Anne Conway was obviously pulling out all the stops and offering the inducement of names and organisations that might entice Frances to join a grand committee. Frances wanted to do her own thing and had not had much response to earlier contacts with RSPCA, SCAS etc. She was already forming her own support group in Kenilworth, but after the advice of her father, who had also consulted me, Frances went down to the London meeting. From later accounts of that meeting, Frances had stuck out for what she wanted: to use rescue and unwanted (abandoned) dogs, and to have two types of dogs trained: the active assistance dog trained to wheelchair users' requirements and 'social dogs' that would offer a less target orientated assistant dog. She had already taken on a dog and placed it in an old persons' home in Kenilworth: an early example of AAI.

It is probable that Frances actually walked out of the London Gwynne Hart meeting when she found the others there had different ideas from her own. She was remonstrated with by one of the organisers as she left but, her mind was made up to go ahead with dog training and avoid working with a large committee based far from Kenilworth.

Dogs for the Disabled had a modest start. Working from a small office in the basement of an end of terrace house, the charity was not registered with the Charity Commission until 1988. Volunteer trainer Jenny Cotton came in to train a German Shepherd that had been donated to Frances. Other helpers were Nicky Philips, a Kenilworth girl, Doreen Cross, the secretarial helper, Denis Fitter, who arranged publicity, and Carolyn Fraser, who later came as a dog trainer from Coventry.

Doreen, who had applied as a helper to Frances, told me her first interview was unconventional; when she rang the doorbell of Frances' house a head popped out of an upstairs window, followed by instructions to let herself in as the door keys were dropped down from above. Doreen said there was no shorthand or typing test, they merely chatted away about the plans and ambitions for a charity. Doreen was then asked if she would start in two days' time. When she asked if there were other applicants for the job to be interviewed, Frances said she always followed her 'gut feeling' about people and reckoned she could do the job.

Doreen started at 9.30 on the Monday, which gave time for Frances to prepare herself for the basement office; she said the Trustees had decided that she must have help in the office. She would then go off for the day, meeting people and leaving Doreen to mind the house. When Frances was away overnight, she had two short stays in hospital, but was then known to discharge herself. Doreen would be asked to feed the cat, attend to the callers, open the post and receive telephone calls. Sometimes there were as many as five dogs in the house. Two, Kim and Misty, were there as demonstrators, while the others were temporary borders.

Although Frances eventually became very ill, Doreen, who came in daily to the house, said she had been determined to keep a hospital appointment in December 1990 and made her way there by taxi. 'How she did this I do not know,' said Doreen. When the hospital saw her condition, they kept her in of course - she died there a few days later. Doreen wrote about this event some years later.

Carolyn said she first heard about Frances in an article in the weekly paper 'Our Dogs'. she was living in Coventry, only a few miles from Kenilworth, and got in touch to offer help. She was taken on and given a free hand to choose and train dogs as an experienced trainer. Carolyn had started training at the Bolton Centre of the Guide Dogs for the Blind in 1970 and eight years later returned to Coventry, married with two boys and a daughter, Faye, who also came along to help. Carolyn found suitable rescue dogs and sometimes unwanted dogs were brought to her own house, where she conducted most of their training.

Shep was one such dog, an alert black and white Collie which was found abandoned, with her pads bleeding, beside a Coventry dual carriageway. Frances wrote at that time: 'The demand for dogs is enormous, not only to give physical help but just as important to give companionship, a sense of independence, like my Kim'. She could also see the benefit of using unwanted or abandoned dogs, especially those deposited in the rescue kennels just outside Coventry. She wrote: 'The concept of saving the lives of many dogs and using them to make life easier and happier for disabled people is one which will pull at the heartstrings of a great many people and many of them will be only too glad to give a donation, be it small or large, to turn the concept into reality'.

To establish a registered charity, a board of Trustees needed to be appointed. The Kenilworth branch of Round Table had offered a solicitor and an accountant to help Frances. The accountant was approached, but she did not stay long, while a solicitor, Ian Burr, became a Trustee early in 1988, followed two months later by myself and John Hall, who Frances introduced as the person who would be her first Chairman of the Trustees' board. I decided to join having seen what a dog could do for Kerry in the USA, on the understanding that it was only necessary to attend the monthly meetings.

Before the charity group became better known, a move away from Kenilworth was forced, only two years after the charity had been registered. Frances' unexpected death in December 1990 required the quick sale of her house. The charity was temporarily homeless, with just two part-time secretaries and no assets. Fortunately amongst those in Frances' small supporters' group was David Wilson, the administrator at the Leamington Guide Dog Centre, who in 1989 had joined as one of the Trustees. He was able to negotiate for the use at a nominal rent of a vacant Portakabin which the new charity could use on the GDBA premises in Leamington.

Frances's aide and secretary Doreen, helped by Linda Crawley, moved into the temporary office, which was already furnished with desks and chairs and a telephone extension from the GDBA switchboard. The one typewriter in use was not so reliable, but with the help of a donation from the local Lions Group, there was enough money left over, after paying debts, for a computer to be purchased for £1000. A copying machine was later donated by Hills Nutrition.

The charity was run on a shoestring, and there was only the one part-time trainer working for Dogs for the Disabled from her Coventry home. With more awareness of the work, two members of GDBA staff volunteered to help with the dog training. They were officially seconded by the larger charity to work to help the newer dog charity Dogs for the Disabled to establish itself. It was felt that working with a different type of dog would enhance their experience and help them to become good trainers of guide dogs (or that was how an arrangement was negotiated at Leamington). Frances' inspiration, as told by her father, was that losing your leg as a teenager might either make one seek a sheltered life or look for ways of making life better for other people who experienced disability problems.

The words of her own father, a much-travelled member of the Diplomatic Service, give a clue to what made this teenager take on a competitive role in her shortened life. He wrote:

'Frances was born on 19th August 1949 in a private Nursing Home in Epsom Surrey to LAC and Dorinne Newns (nee Dryden). The entire family (self, wife, three children - sons aged eight and six) went to Delhi in the autumn of 1953. The boys went to boarding school in the hills. Frances, then only 4 years old, was too young for school. We were transferred to Madras in 1955. We put the boys in boarding school in the UK. Frances came with us and started in the kindergarten class of a school run by the Presentation Convent. She was then six years old. The convent also had a boarding school for older girls in Kodai Kanal, a hill station in the Nilgiri Hills some 400 miles from Madras. After a year or two Frances transferred to that school.

'We were next transferred to Singapore in 1961, where for the benefit of the armed forces stationed there, the Alexandra Secondary Modern School had been set up. Frances went to that school. She was then 11, coming up to 12 years old. We were living in Singapore till 1964 and had two periods of UK leave in that time, when Frances was placed temporarily in UK state schools. From Singapore we were transferred to Adelaide, South Australia, where Frances at 15 years of age was placed in Muirden College, a commercial finishing school for girls.

'Not long after she started at that college, a painful swelling appeared on the left side of her left leg just below the knee. It was kept under observation by our GP, but instead of increasing in size it subsided and resumed normal size. Then one day, when she was waiting for a bus to take her to the college a brick-laden lorry passed the bus stop and shed one of its bricks, which struck Frances on the place where the swelling had previously occurred. It was a painful experience and tragically the swelling re-appeared and this time did not subside. In due course X-rays and subsequent biopsies revealed cancer of the tibia.

'The specialist called in my wife and me to tell us of the diagnosis and his first words were 'I'm afraid you've got to resign yourselves to the fact that the leg has got to come off'. But first it (the cancer) had to be killed and for that she had to have immediate radiology. The method used was to put her in a tube under four atmospheres of pressure twice a week for three weeks. [I had been given two choices. One was to have radiotherapy every day for about 6 weeks or the pressurised treatment that I chose]. The specialists then referred me to Sir Stamford Cade, a Harley Street specialist, regarded at the time as the leading expert on cancer. I arranged to take immediate leave and my wife and I travelled to London with Fran. At this point of time Fran was wearing a calliper on her leg, because the radiology treatment had significantly weakened the bones in the leg. What she didn't know was that the doctors in Adelaide had told us that cancer of the bone almost invariably settled in the pulmonary area, which would be fatal, and that this could happen within two years.

'Sir Stamford Cade carried out his own tests and arranged further radiotherapy treatment over six weeks at Westminster hospital and got us to agree a date for the amputation. After the treatment he pronounced that the cancer was dead, and that there was no sign of it in the lungs.

'Though Sir Stamford Cade was in private practice, he arranged for the amputation to be done at Westminster Hospital under the National Health by a surgeon of his choice, Mr Westbury. We were advised not to tell Fran anything until the night before the operation. So every day for six weeks, I drove Fran to Westminster Hospital from Bounds Green, North London, where we were staying with my wife's parents. After the treatments, we sometimes went into Richmond Park to feed the deer, which made the day for Fran in view of her love of animals.

'As the day of the operation drew near I arranged with the hospital staff that I would go there on the evening before to tell Fran what was going to happen. But when it came to the point I couldn't bring myself to do it and the hospital doctor did it for me. He told me later that all Fran said was 'I think I knew it'.

'The operation took place in the summer of 1965. Sir Stamford Cade inspected the stump and pronounced it 'a beautiful operation' (he himself died only a few years later). After the operation I saw Fran through the first stages of the fitting of her artificial leg, a process which took place in the limb fitting centre in Roehampton (conveniently close to Richmond Park and the deer; incidentally where Douglas

Bader, the war hero, was fitted with his artificial limbs). I then returned to my duties in Adelaide. My wife remained in the UK until Fran was properly fitted with a leg and a spare. They then returned to Adelaide. Frances did not return to her college. Far from seeking a sheltered life, she remained very active and as far as was humanly possible she did all the things a teenager would want to do. She went riding, swimming and even ice skating. She was considered one of Roehampton's star patients and was always ready to try out any new designs of artificial legs, even making a video there to demonstrate her mobility to other patients. Then came her courtship, marriage and with her new husband mingled actively with their friends. It was not until a more mature age that the idea of actively helping others entered her head and the inspiration was solely and entirely due to her dog Kim.

'We returned to the UK in 1968 and lived for a time in Dulwich. Fran got an administrative job in a firm supplying drink dispensing machines, a post which she held until we were transferred to Birmingham, when we took up residence in Hampton-in Arden. Fran got a job as office supervisor with a firm in Sheldon, a post she held until she was married to J C Hay (a dental surgeon) in 1975. Deborah was born in 1977. A few years later Fran was divorced and moved first to Balsall Common, then to London and finally to Kenilworth. In London, when Deborah went to school, Fran took a part-time office job.

'Fran conceived DFD in 1986. Her original idea was to use 'rescue dogs'. She would be giving the dogs a good home and would bring a new life and hope for disabled people (a double benefit). The first thing Fran did was to ring up Central TV in Birmingham and tell them of her idea. It caught their imagination. They sent a news team to visit her. The next major event was a call from Derek Jameson to invite her to his morning radio programme, which had quite a wide audience. On the same programme Jameson had the head of RSPCA to give comments on Fran's scheme. He wasn't particularly supportive and he appeared lost for ideas about dogs being used to help disabled persons.

'There was a lot of public interest following the first TV programme and the letters turned into a flood after the Jameson radio programme. There was very little cash offered, but there were requests for the charity to train the enquirer's own dog, requests for trained Dogs for the Disabled people or their associated groups – one as far away as the Shetlands. There were many offers of people who wanted to supply unwanted dogs, as well as requests to give talks, which in many ways delayed Fran, working on her own from home, in getting the first dog out nearly two years later.

'One of the listeners of the programme was Anne Conway, who immediately got in touch with Fran. She had telephoned and Fran was surprised to learn that a dog training scheme was already planned elsewhere. Anne Conway sent her a large dossier of the information she had assembled on assistance dogs, as at the time she had got quite a long way into her negotiations with the organisers of the assistance dog scheme in Holland and also with Bonita Bergin, the power behind the American equivalent. After that Fran was invited to a meeting in London organised by the PR organisation Graylings. It was thought that Pedigree Chum, a leading dog food brand at that time, was sponsoring Anne Conway. Fran was asked to go as an 'adviser' but after discussing it with me (during the course of which I had a word with you on the phone), she decided she would go to the meeting but only if they accepted her as 'founder'. They agreed to this arrangement, since Fran had started her idea of assistance dogs without outside help.

'Fran found that Anne Conway's ideas were to build up an organisation and a breeding and training centre. Anne Conway was dead against using rescue dogs. As a matter of interest, the RSPCA were at the meeting; Fran thought they were quite indecisive. Fran thought them all long-winded and thought Anne Conway's scheme would take too long to get going, and she decided to paddle her own canoe. Her intention was to get dogs out and to build training centres later. In actual fact it took her nearly two years to get the first trained dog out as she was fully occupied with requests for speeches, telephone and written enquiries, media interviews, putting up displays at sales of work, dog shows etc and other forms of fundraising.

'As she was leaving the London meeting, one of the organisers took her to one side and said 'In our experience, when two new charities set out to achieve the same thing, one of them inevitably fails'. These words merely fired Fran to make a success of her idea, although later the use of rescued dogs had to be phased out.

'In those early days, Fran and her 'Advisory Committee' of loyal friends had the idea that there could be two sorts of Dogs for the Disabled people; well-trained good natured companion dogs; and highly-trained working dogs. To show the world that the charity really was working at this idea, she found and placed in an old persons' home a terrier cross called Holly, which was a great success, and got her some publicity. However the idea of companion dogs had to be dropped since animal assisted therapy (AAT) was harder to 'sell' to the public when fundraising.

'Many of the donated dogs were found to have unreliable temperaments, which did not show up until more demands were made from the dogs as task training was required. Another limiting factor was the availability of trainers; Fran had a natural ability for this but did not have enough experience. Eventually, I think out of her association with dog clubs, Jenny Cotton as a volunteer came along from Coventry, as the first assistance dog trainer used by Fran. Frances' first client. I don't know what motivated Fran to pick Gladys Rainbow from a host of others as the first DFD client but having chosen her, she and Jenny Cotton scoured rescue centres for a suitable dog and eventually chose Rani. They agreed that Jenny should take Rani over and feed and keep her in her home (at the charity's expense) whilst under training. It would have been impracticable otherwise. Fran was able to pay Jenny a small fee for the work. Gladys Rainbow was trained to use the dog in her own home in Rugby. Amongst other things, Rani had to be conditioned to the use of a wheelchair. Jenny Cotton made a good job of training Rani but declined to take on any more dogs.

'Fran decided to aim to stage a major event for the handing over of Rani to Gladys Rainbow. She persuaded a PR firm in Kenilworth to deal with the media free of charge, and got the Kenilworth De Montfort hotel to provide a large reception area plus refreshments (all for nothing). And she got the mayor of Kenilworth to make the presentation. It was a very successful operation. David Wilson came from the guide dog charity and his presence was to have unforeseen benefits later. The De Montfort continued to support Fran in quite a handsome way. Trustees' meetings were held in one of their reception rooms when the group became too large for Fran's house.

'I can't remember when you, Dick, joined our forces, but you probably know as much about the subsequent dogs as I do. But I think the next two dog partnerships were Amanda Coplans with Poppy and Gina Geary with Ben. Both were London based. They had a big spread in Woman's Own and Amanda was featured, with Fran present, on Blue Peter children's TV. Deborah had produced the Woman's Own article, which also mentioned a child, Abigail Slater, and her newly-trained dog Marty. All these dogs were trained by Caroline Fraser, who had by then taken on the role of head trainer. She worked from her home in Coventry and helped by her daughter Fay, was dedicated to giving the dogs the right start.

'Frances' own assistance dog Kim was a rescue dog. She had weak back legs and had pancreas trouble. Trust Fran to take pity on disabled dogs! Misty (Siberian Husky type) was also a rescue dog. Amie (Golden Retriever) was donated by a breeder as a puppy and was named by children from a local school. Misty and Amie, when she was older, accompanied Fran on her many speeches as demonstration dogs. Fran's very first dog (a Border Collie cross which we called Nicky) had been found by her brother abandoned in a monsoon ditch in Delhi, and remained with us throughout our sojourns in Madras and Singapore. In her time Fran had a variety of pets. Dogs, cats, a tortoise, a white mouse, a parrot and tropical fish. She had a love of animals of all kinds and this was mentioned in her school reports. She was an outstandingly good athlete, swimmer and horse rider and won several prizes and trophies in all three sports: in Madras (as a junior rider) and in Singapore (swimming and running). In Singapore she won the school Junior sportsmanship trophy in 1963 and represented the school in a number of sporting activities. She had a natural talent for painting. All of her paintings were of animals.'

Frances as Director General

There was a need to have the name 'Dogs for the Disabled' registered at the Charity Commission as a charity for assistance dogs. Frances assumed the Director's title, and she had appointed a dog friend as the first chairman of her group; Ernie Lester from the local area attended the first meetings with a few Kenilworth supporters and Fran's father. With the intention of registering the charity, an invitation was made to any interested person to become a Trustee. One of these supporters who was active in the first year was a dog trainer who had worked as a handyman at the Leamington GDBA kennels; unfortunately when it came to registering persons as Trustees, his name was unexpectedly withdrawn, as a past incident on record made him unsuitable. Ian Burr, the solicitor, and I, as well as John Hall who was to be the next Chairman joined as Trustees in 1988. My first meeting with Frances a year earlier was when I went to a gathering that was held in the bar of a Kenilworth pub, the Gauntlet, in May 1987. Rani, a German Shepherd dog in training, was introduced to some of the 50 invited supporters present that evening, but there was an apparent lack of any real organisation. Frances spoke at the bar about her plans to train more dogs, but parts of her speech were drowned by the pub's music system. It was a start in forming the new charity.

Two more dogs, Ben and Poppy, were trained after Rani, using a new trainer in the next year. A limited company had already been set up for trading purposes as Dogs for the Disabled, but the formalities of an organisation that the charity commissioners would accept still had to be completed. An advisory committee for the charity, with 10 persons, first met on October 20th 1988 in Kenilworth; Caroline Fraser, an experienced dog trainer, and Gina Geary, who had already been trained with German Shepherd Ben, represented the dog side. Others who came along had professional experience, while others had been helping by collecting money or attending at dog shows. Frances not only selected those to help her but also personally interviewed and chose the persons who might be suited to an available dog, Ann Greenwood in Cornwall being such a person. Through telephone contact only, she was able to have a dog sent to her together with a trainer who was working far from her home. The charity became registered in 1989 (with the Charity Commission number 700454). Once a set of audited accounts had been sent in the structure of the group with officers and Trustees had been agreed.

In May of that year, the new but struggling charity made a first approach to Julian Oxley, the Secretary and Director of Administration at the guide dog charity, with a request for some form of support. At this point Dogs for the Disabled, with no publicity, had a waiting list of 15 people with various disabilities, and each had completed application forms to have dogs. There was only the one part-time trainer available, who was then fully occupied training a single dog for the child in Chester, so the situation was critical. The income of about £1000 a month from fundraising was erratic and not sufficient to pay wages for a second trainer.

It was natural to turn to a much wealthier local dog training charity for help. The guide dog training organisation (GDBA) was already well established in Warwickshire, having been relocated to Leamington in 1940 during the early stages of World War II. Their 1930s training base and their kennels at Wallasey near Liverpool were made unusable when an anti-aircraft gun site was placed next door in 1939 and started letting off practice rounds! Captain Liakhof, head of the GDBA, urgently searched for a new location to train dogs in a safer area. It was said that as the GWR rail route from London to Birkenhead stopped at Leamington, he chose to look there as a safe town, and after a short search he had been able to move into an old riverside property, Edmonscote Manor. He was a pioneer trainer of guide dogs, but his 'apprentice' once told me that hitting the dog's head onto the wing of a car was a method employed to make a dog realise cars could cause pain. Fortunately punishment was no longer used as a method of reinforcement.

The location was ideal, with extensive grounds around an old manor house that extended down to the River Leam. The GDBA were fortunate enough to own a site that gave room for expansion for kennel blocks and car parking as the demand for guide dogs increased. There had been an earlier meeting between Fran and her solicitor, together with David Wilson representing the Guide Dogs for the Blind Association, who had recently been appointed as the Leamington Administrator. David had a commercial background, having worked in the motor industry in the Philippines amongst other things, selling Leyland buses. He had a greater interest in developing new facilities, unlike many in the GDBA who only knew about training dogs with blind people, which was enough of a challenge.

David had noticed the publicity that Fran was receiving in the media and he said he would further the idea that GDBA's skill with guide dogs could be used to help by offering general advice on setting up the organisation and giving advice on how to train dogs. Also considered was the possible use of spare GDBA kennel space; they could provide for the loan of stands for publicity at fetes and open air shows, and best of all possibly even to supply suitable dogs.

He urged Frances to write to the Director General of the GDBA stating her plans. It was fortunate that the person at the top was Major General John Groom, recently retired RE engineer from the Army. His previous job had been to hasten the building of runways in the Falkland Isles; he was a forceful character but based away from Warwickshire at the Windsor GDBA head office. He too had a more worldly outlook on the use of dogs and possibly would have seen the military dogs at work in the Royal Army Veterinary Corps units overseas. Unlike others he did not consider it a threat to the established GDBA charity that a new but tiny charity would want to train dogs near to the Leamington GDBA centre. Initially he was very supportive but later there seemed to be a cooling off, and it was even suggested that someone mistook General Groom's interest and with his name linked him to another old and well established London-based registered charity known as 'John Groom's Crippleage'. This was entirely untrue, but it was used derisively by certain persons indoctrinated by the idea that dogs could only guide the blind. Suggesting it was a waste of money to train dogs for any other purpose, they started speaking out against the idea. The London disability charity later changed its name to one with a more politically correct title.

The GDBA had to be careful not to antagonise its supporters by diverting funds to another charity not associated with blindness, although other ways could be found to give a degree of support. Blind persons growing older might need wheelchairs, and diabetics who lost their sight sometimes had to have parts of their limbs amputated in consequence of the disease. The request made for the GDBA to help Dogs for the Disabled in 1989 was successful. It was agreed that two seconded dog training staff would be made available. At first they were used on a temporary basis for developing the idea to convert some of the dogs which were unsuitable for guide dog work to becoming 'helping dogs for wheelchair users' or 'other handicapped persons'. The letter to the Director General of the GDBA had been drafted by Frances' father, and after it was amended it was sent carrying my own signature, D Lane, as I had by then been elected Chairman of the Trustees.

Once the application was accepted favourably, Dogs for the Disabled charity would again move forward with its development plans. Fundraising would remain entirely separate from any help GDBA provided to the charity, and that was the next challenge for the board of Trustees to face.

Chapter 3

Anne Conway and Canine Partners' Development

Whilst Dogs for the Disabled was progressing slowly in the 1990s and overcoming various setbacks, in the south of England a charity with many similar aims was operating under the guidance of Anne Conway. Frances Hay had been intent on getting dogs trained and placed with disabled persons from the outset. She may have known her life would be shorter than others, and the need to fulfil her expectations of her canine charity, producing assistance dogs as soon as possible, was her main concern.

In 1987 there had been an exchange of communications between Anne and Frances. Archived letter dated 24/2/87 To Anne Conway:

I have now blossomed into some headed notepaper and have designed a logo for the scheme. The dog in the logo is an exact replica of Kim and will be what I hope is a permanent memento of the fact that it was she who first started me off on this scheme. I still miss her very much, even though Misty, her replacement, is such a joy to me. I have been so immersed in all the work that has arisen from the development of the scheme that I have not been able to pause to take stock of how far I have got. But I have now made myself do this and have prepared a summary of the progress I have made and, quite honestly, it is as much a surprise to me as it will probably be to others. At least the scheme has not yet failed as a result of lack of organisational planning, as apparently happened to that poor young man in Devon Stuart has told us about.

For my own part, I wonder whether the cause of his demise of his ideas was not so much his organising ability as possibly he didn't get the positive support he needed. I perhaps have been luckier for, as you will see from my summary of progress, a copy of which I am enclosing, I have received tremendous active and financial support from a lot of local organisations. To tell you the truth, now that I have taken stock of where I have got to, I am seriously beginning to wonder whether the committee we have had in mind right from the outset of the scheme is really going to get further along the road of progress than I've managed to achieve under my own steam. This is not to say I think I know it all, or that I didn't make mistakes, or couldn't do things a better way, and I really am anxious to get as much benefit as I can from people experienced in this sort of thing or who have professional expertise. But do I really need a committee for that? Can you see in what specific ways such a committee might help? Might they not just delay things a bit? I must say that right at the beginning I felt a real need for guidance on many of the points that were bothering me then (and which I detailed in my suggestion of an Agenda for the first meeting) are gradually getting answered as I forge along my pragmatic path. In any case if such a committee eventually materialised perhaps it ought to be held up here, where all the action is taking place. Furthermore I feel it would only be fair that my present financial Sponsors should be closely associated with it.

'All in all, my own feeling is that I should continue as I have been going, at least for the time being. I have very much appreciated your own help and encouragement and am particularly grateful for the unstinting way in which you furnished me with all the information at your disposal. And I hope we can continue that relationship in the future. I do not wish to slam the door on the committee proposal. It just doesn't seem very opportune at this moment in time.

Frances Hay (Mrs)

A copy of this letter had gone to Stuart Hutton, who was also trying to coordinate setting up assistance dog training in his role as Chairman of the Society for Companion Animal Studies (SCAS). The proposed committee was never formed; eventually a coordinating group, Assistance Dogs (UK), would be set up many years later. Following the Grayling 1988 meeting in London, Frances and Anne agreed to go their own separate ways. Anne's house in Hampshire became her base for her charity, Assistance Dogs for the Disabled People. Registered in the same year as Dogs for the Disabled, their assistance dog training developed more slowly, so that their first group of dogs were not issued until June 1994.

I am grateful to Rosemary Smith, who was at the heart of Canine Partners development, for this account of the difficulties then successes in starting a charity:

'During the 1980s, dogs were getting a bad press, which concerned Anne Conway greatly. Throughout her life she had shown a great love for dogs and had built up quite a reputation for her responsible and expert handling and training of them. She owned cocker spaniels and understood them well. It was her belief that the problems being reported in the press were caused by irresponsible ownership and in her view this was unfair on the dogs. Such was her interest in the animals and the bond between humans and dogs that she went to the

Delta conference on dog behaviour and the human/animal bond held in America and run by Bonita Bergin, who was heavily involved with Canine Companions for Independence (CCI).

'Anne learned how the charity was training dogs to assist disabled people to gain greater independence. At the conference she met Liz Ormerod, a vet who was practising in the north east of England, and they both came away very impressed with the results of the work in the States. Anne believed that if such a charity existed in England it would help improve the public image of the dog, whilst at the same time providing valuable help to disabled people. She returned to England excited by what she had learned and set about talking to the many contacts she had made in the dog world in the hope that she could persuade someone to start such a charity in England, but there were no takers. In the end she realised that if her ideas were to get off the ground then she would have to start the charity herself.

'Punctilious in everything she did, Anne set about researching how to set up and fund a charity, what breeds of dogs would be most suited to such work, what training would be required and what types of disability would be likely to benefit most. Her research was incredibly thorough, taking her far and wide across the world. She read everything she could lay her hands on, she talked with many of the experts working in the various disciplines involved and she left no stone unturned in the pursuit of her aims. She talked to doctors, occupational therapists, disabled people themselves, vets, dog trainers, charity workers and managers, fundraisers, the Charity Commission, solicitors, in fact anyone who could help her in one or other aspect of starting up such a complex charity.

'Eventually her travels took her to Holland, where she visited SOHO, a Dutch charity which had already started training Dogs for the Disabled people. She was extremely impressed with their method of training the dogs and decided that their work would be the blueprint for her charity. There were certain aspects about the actual training of the dogs in the States which she did not like, and she found the more gentle practice of praise and reward carried out in the Netherlands much more to her liking.

'Nearing the end of her research into assistance dogs, she heard a programme on BBC Radio Two in which Derek Jameson was interviewing Frances Hay on a charity she was setting up in Kenilworth called Dogs for the Disabled. Realising that the aims of the charity matched her own, Anne was quick to spot the potential in the two charities joining together with pooled resources, and she telephoned Frances to discuss the matter. Through her contacts in Pedigree Petfoods, Anne succeeded in getting a meeting set up in London at the offices of Grayling, the PR agents of Pedigree, who were also of the view that there should be only one charity. Unfortunately the meeting did not go well due to the fundamental differences in temperament and personality of Frances Hay and Anne Conway. Anne's approach was measured, thorough, long ranging and academic, as opposed to Frances, who was looking at the situation from an emotional point of view; having lost a leg due to cancer and realising the help her own pet dog could give her, she wanted to get things off the ground immediately. Entirely opposite to Anne, who wanted absolutely everything to be in place before she even started to train a dog. There was simply no common ground between them, and Frances left the meeting.

'Realising that she was on her own, once her research was complete Anne set about the all-important task of getting the charity registered with the Charity Commission and set up as a company limited by guarantee and registered at Companies House. The Memorandum and Articles of Association were based on those in use in the Guide Dogs for the Blind Association and Hearing Dogs for the Deaf, a charity for which she was a Trustee. She called her charity

Assistance Dogs for the Disabled People, having ascertained that many disabled people disliked being lumped together under the generic term 'the disabled'. The paper she presented to the Charity Commission was superb in its detail. It covered every conceivable aspect of the work of the charity. Nothing had been left unconsidered and not researched. It was a masterpiece and for many years following provided the backcloth for all that happened in the charity. When in doubt the answer would always be found in her paper. Charity registration was granted on 27 June 1990 and the company was registered at Companies House at much the same time.

'Her next job was to find a group of people from various backgrounds who would be prepared to act as Trustees of the charity and help get it off the ground. She recruited a vet, an occupational therapist, a disabled person, a dog trainer, a solicitor, a bookkeeper and a rheumatologist as well as two people from the world of business.

'The Trustee meetings were initially all held in Anne's house in Hampshire. She personally funded the setting up of the charity and did all the secretarial work herself, obviously on a voluntary basis. She had already managed to raise some funds and she guarded the purse strings with enormous care. She was not ready to spend one penny of the charitable funds raised from her own endeavours and those of various volunteers. The Trustees realised that whilst it would be nice to achieve utopia before actually starting to train dogs, realistically funds would never come in in sufficient quantity until there were dogs out on the street working with disabled people and the public could see for themselves the benefit to the disabled people. This was agreed and the search was on to find a Trainer sufficiently qualified to train assistance dogs.

'Advertisements were placed and applications came in. Anne shortlisted those she considered could be suitable and set up an interviewing panel which included herself and Tony Blunt, the Chief Executive of Hearing Dogs for the Deaf. They selected Nina Bondarenko, an Australian who had a great deal of experience training, handling and judging dogs in her home country where she was brought up with Rottweilers. Even as a child Nina was interested in the animal mind and set about trying to understand how the dogs thought and reacted to her commands. By the time she came over to England she was particularly interested in the human-animal bond and the opportunity to join a new charity training dogs to assist disabled people was of particular interest to her and she soon settled down to devise the training programme. In 1992, once she had agreed a way forward, she visited various breeders and selected four Golden Retriever puppies which she called Amos, Alfred, Angus and Alex. At the same time she found four willing volunteers to take the puppies into their homes socialise them and start them on their training under Nina's guidance. The charity rented a house for Nina out in the Hampshire countryside and she moved in, meeting the puppy walkers on a regular basis, when she checked the development of the puppies and trained them towards their future role as assistance dogs.

'The puppies' health was looked after by John Whitaker at his veterinary practice in Hampshire. He became so interested in the charity that he treated the dogs at a discount and became a Trustee. Anne Conway was still heavily involved with all the administrative work and fundraising and it was agreed that an administrator be recruited to share the burden. Mrs Chilton joined the charity and worked in an office near Chichester. It was not easy for her as she was completely on her own and it was not easy for Anne to give over her cherished work. The charity was, after all, her baby. Despite this, things worked out reasonably well at first.

'The Trustees were keen to learn as much as possible about running a business and invited a management consultant in for a day's training. One outcome from this day was a decision that the name of the charity, Assistance Dogs for the Disabled People, was a bit of a mouthful and not readily understood by the public. At the time the charity was divided into two committees. The Canine Committee, chaired by John Whitaker, the vet, was responsible for the welfare and training of the dogs, and the other was headed up by Roddy Russell, an Occupational Therapist and that committee was responsible for the selection of recipients for the dogs. They called themselves the ADAPT Committee. This stood for Assistance Dogs and People Together. The Trustees agreed that this would be an excellent name for the charity and this change of name was registered with the Charity Commission.

'Ultimately, however, this proved to be a disastrous decision. In 1989 the powerful Carnegie Trust had realised that the majority of arts venues were inaccessible to disabled people and, convinced of the rights of disabled people to share in the arts, they set up the ADAPT Fund (Access for Disabled people to Arts Premises Today). The founders wished to challenge venue owners and managers to think about essential improvements and to plan to fund these from their own resources, augmented, if approved, by the ADAPT Fund. Carnegie offered to start the fund with £250,000, on condition that that sum could be matched from other sources. When the Carnegie Trustees discovered that a small charity was calling itself ADAPT they objected and asked that the name be changed (ADAPT was also used by a domestic abuser charity set up in Ireland in 1974). Having just changed the name, not surprisingly, the Trustees were resistant to the thought of another name change and they decided to take on the Carnegie Trust, bearing in mind that their charity had formerly been registered with the Charity Commission. David Carrick and several Trustees from the charity attended a meeting with members of the Carnegie Trust in the House of Commons, but the Carnegie Trust would not give an inch.

They held firm, and realising that they could not afford a legal fight, David and his colleagues had no choice but to give in very reluctantly.

'The following months were incredibly difficult because the charity had no name so could not fundraise, and with no name, it had no headed paper, so communication was impossible. It really was a very black time for the charity. Eventually, bearing in mind the American charity Canine Companions for Independence (CCI), Liz Ormerod, one of the Trustees, suggested that the charity be called Canine Partners for Independence, with the acronym CPI. A sense of relief invaded the Trustees' meeting as this suggestion was adopted.

'Anne immediately set about getting the new name registered and getting the headed paper printed. It was also agreed that professional fundraisers be engaged to give the fundraising a real boost. It had been stagnant for far too long and things were looking bleak. The fundraisers were engaged and succeeded in getting Lord Harewood to agree to be the Patron. This was a great start. As cousin to the Queen, his involvement with the charity would give it real authority, and excitement was brewing amongst the Trustees, but it was to be short-lived. The fundraisers held a fundraising event in London to which Nina took the puppies and Lord Harewood attended. It was a financial disaster and in the end the Fundraisers cost the charity some £26,500 and raised just a few hundred pounds. The financial year to June 1993 ended with a deficit of £45,550. The Fundraisers went bankrupt. Sadly it was necessary to dispense with the services of the Administrator and close the office, but the Chairman of the charity, an accountant working in London, agreed that his offices could be used for an Administrator and one was engaged, but even worse was to follow.

'Whilst at work one day, the Administrator was horrified to be faced with the bailiffs, who had come to seize the assets of the Chairman as, unbeknown to the charity, his accountancy business had folded and was in serious trouble. She managed to hold on to the few

43

possessions which belonged to CPI and these were transferred back down to Anne. There was no choice but to dispense with her services, as she had nowhere to work and she felt she would be better off finding another job.

'By February 1994, with only some £7,000 in the bank and debts of some £13,000, things were really looking bleak and at a Trustee meeting some of the Trustees felt that the charity should be closed. Anne was demoralised by the turn of events and felt that the charity was simply not meant to be and could not continue. The Chairman resigned and it looked like the end. However there is always hope and Rosemary Smith, Trustee, felt a strong responsibility towards those volunteers and supporters who had helped and put money into the charity. She felt strongly that they should not be let down and said that if the Trustees were prepared to give her their backing and elect her Chairman and give her some freedom, she would do everything in her power to get the charity back on its feet, but if she had not succeeded within 12 months, then there really would be no choice but to close. As this was the only offer on the table other than immediate closure, the Trustees agreed and Rosemary Smith was duly elected Chairman.

'Her first job was to ensure that the puppies whose puppy training was now complete would have somewhere to be housed and trained for the advanced part of their training. A meeting was set up at Anne's house, where she generously offered her late mother's house, Kingsey House, as a training centre for the dogs and a home for Nina on a short-term lease. Her offer was accepted with alacrity. The house was close by and was a very old house with a good-sized garden. There was plenty of room for the four dogs and Nina moved in with them. Some of the Trustees erected a gate so that the dogs would be safe. It was not the most comfortable of homes but Nina did sterling work training the dogs for their future roles.

'Having got the dogs on course, Rosemary's next task was to get some volunteers to run the administrative side of the charity. Several signed up and were allocated a room in the house, although it was necessary to get a change of planning permission to run an office there. David Carrick, Trustee, saw this through. It was not easy for the volunteers as there was no immediate supervision and Rosemary was working full time many miles away in Berkshire but they did a good job in very difficult circumstances.

'Inevitably the next job for Rosemary was to get the fundraising back on track. Through Roger Jefcoate, Vice President, she was introduced to a company which was a member of the Association of Fundraising Consultants and who helped charities raise funds through Charitable Trusts. Before a meeting could be arranged with Keith Davison from the company, she discovered that the previous Chairman had run up a large bill with a London firm of solicitors and it had not been paid. He had engaged these solicitors to represent the charity when the Carnegie Trust asked that the name of the charity be changed. They were now suing the charity for payment, as the Chairman had not answered any of their letters nor responded to any of their telephone calls. At the same time as she discovered this problem she learned that the Home Office was not prepared to extend Nina's work permit. Realising that she was getting out of her depth Rosemary decided to telephone a contact she had been given in Guide Dogs for the Blind whose Head Office was close to her home. She wanted to ask them for some advice, but they were not able to help and no meeting was arranged. Fortunately Rosemary relished a challenge and feeling passionate about the aims of the charity and a responsibility towards all those who had helped and supported the charity, she decided to meet the problems head on. She was also being very ably supported by some of the Trustees.

'David Carrick set up a meeting with the local MP to discuss Nina's work permit. He was very sympathetic to the case, realising that Nina was fundamental to the success of the charity. Apart from Frances Hay's charity Dogs for the Disabled, there were no other charities in England training dogs to assist disabled people. Nina was the expert, and irreplaceable. Following the MP's advice, David succeeded in getting Nina a six-month extension to her work permit, but it was made clear that there would be no further extension.

'Despite the stay of execution being so short, Rosemary turned her mind to dealing with the solicitor's unpaid bill. After some difficulty she ascertained the name, address and telephone number of the solicitor the previous Chairman had dealt with and rang him up. She sensed relief in his voice when she introduced herself and a meeting was arranged in London. As she drove up she had no clear idea as to how she would approach the matter. The charity owed the solicitors several thousand pounds which it did not have, and somehow she had to come away from the meeting with a deal that would satisfy both sides and withdrawal of the legal action which already had a date for hearing. They met and a rapport was established. The solicitor was brilliant, and agreed to withdraw action on the basis that the charity pay some two thirds of the total bill over a period of three months with equal payments each month and the remaining third written off. Knowing a good deal when she saw one, Rosemary accepted and left with the solicitor's words ringing in her ears: 'You fight a hard corner'.

'Needless to say she wrote and thanked him profusely, the money was paid as agreed, the debt settled and the legal action withdrawn. CPI then discovered that the Treasurer had not been paying in any National Insurance Contributions for the Administrator and for Nina and CPI not only had all the back payments to make but an excess had been levied for late payment. What a nightmare! Rosemary managed to raise £1,000 from a sale held in her garden and that helped, but it was now imperative that she met with Keith Davison to discuss Charitable Trust funding. They met at her home during her lunch break from her own employment. She will never forget Keith's face when she told him of the problems facing the charity. The blood simply drained away and he went as white as a sheet. She laughed and told him not to worry, as she would sort everything out if he could put her in contact with Charitable Trusts, which he did. He sent her a list of all the names and addresses of Charitable Trusts who helped disabled people and Rosemary wrote to every one of them.

'The Treasurer resigned and one of the Trustees, Ray Tidbury, recommended that Dennis Howard be appointed in his place. Dennis duly joined CPI and the Trustees could now relax knowing that the accounts were in excellent hands. He had his eye on the ball, was totally trustworthy, was keenly interested in the work of the charity and kept the books superbly well. He also lived in Hampshire.

'It was at this point that a letter was received from Lord Harewood to the effect that he was not impressed with the management of the charity and was considering his position. Rosemary managed to get some time off work to meet with him at his London flat and was joined there by David Carrick. Between them they persuaded his Lordship that the charity was now under new management and they were doing their utmost to get it back on track. He agreed to stay with the charity and Rosemary promised to keep him in touch with developments. This was the first of several meetings Rosemary had with the Earl over the next few years. His support was superb and the relationship between them became strong. There developed a mutual trust which she treasured.

'In the meantime Nina was continuing to train the four puppies, who were doing well. A new application was being prepared to obtain permanent residency for her and David Carrick was again in contact with the MP over this. Subsequently Nina engaged the services of a barrister who had been recommended to her as he specialised in work permit applications. It was agreed that the charity would help pay his fee, which was not insubstantial. By the end of the financial year, in June 1994, the horrendous loss of the previous year had been turned into a small profit of some £7,000. Over £20,000 had been received from Charitable Trusts and this was making a big difference to the income of the Charity. Suddenly the Trustees began to think that the charity might get through after all and a mood of optimism invaded the camp.

'The Recipient Committee found four disabled recipients for the dogs but unfortunately one of them dropped out at the last minute and there was insufficient time to find a replacement. It was therefore agreed that Amos would remain with his puppy walker, where he had a wonderful life living near the sea with a family who adored him. For Rosemary there was a sadness that he was not placed because it was her own group of voluntary supporters in Wokingham who had raised the £5,000 to sponsor him, but she kept in touch with him for the rest of his life and knew he was happy.

'Three senior members of the SOHO Foundation in Holland, CPI's mentor organisation, came over to assess the dogs, as it was felt essential to have the dogs evaluated by impartial experts in the field as to their suitability to proceed to the next stage of their training, the two-week recipient training course, where the dogs and disabled people are trained together. Fortunately all four dogs passed this assessment.

'Nina, with Roddy Russell, the Occupational Therapist and Trustee, launched the two-week residential course in a residential house for disabled people in Bracklesham Bay in August 1994. Both Roddy and Nina put a great deal of effort and hard work into planning the course, setting out the aims and objectives, raising a teaching plan and writing the support material. Nina had also arranged for Channel Four to film a documentary whilst the course was in progress as this would give tremendous publicity for the charity. The three recipients were all severely physically disabled and all in wheelchairs. They had been carefully selected bearing in mind their background, need, living environment and ability to control and exercise the dog. Despite the difficulties of having a film crew ever present and electric leads trailing across carpets, so potentially hazardous to wheelchairs, all three entered with gusto into the spirit of the training. There was so much to learn but they showed such grit and determination to achieve their ambition to pass the tests and go home with their dog. The dogs and recipients had been carefully matched and the hard work put in by all concerned paid off when all three dogs and recipients came through the course with flying colours. Graduation Day was on Friday 26th August 1994. At 3 pm the graduation ceremony took place in front of the families and friends of the recipients, the puppy walkers who had trained and socialised the puppies, the Trustees of the charity, supporters and volunteers and some local dignitaries and of course Channel Four was there to televise the proceedings.

'As each recipient was called forward to receive their graduation certificate, Nina gave a heartwarming account of their struggles during the course and their determination to succeed. Anne spoke about her delight that she had achieved what she had desired for so long. It was a very moving occasion. The lives of all three recipients were enriched and they became inveterate fundraisers for the charity. The dogs seemed to enjoy their work immensely and the bond which developed between dog and person became incredibly strong.

'What few people at the ceremony knew was that just before the course was due to take place Dennis, the Treasurer, telephoned Rosemary to tell her that the funds were dwindling below an acceptable level and he had no choice but to recommend foreclosure and asked her to take the appropriate action. So worried was he that he rang more than once! There was only enough money to survive another two weeks normal operation. Although she knew that CPI could not even afford the costs of the course she also knew that those dogs had to be placed and desperately wanting the charity to succeed, she wrote to every Charitable Trust she could get hold of to raise funds. At the same time she arranged for the two trainers from Dogs for the Disabled to attend the Recipient Training Course, on the understanding that if she failed to raise the necessary cash then they would take the recipients and dogs over and look after their aftercare. This they agreed to do. The gods must have been smiling on the charity at that time, because in the middle of the course Rosemary received a cheque for £40,000 from a Trust to which she had just written. The Trust was closing down and gave the charity the remaining balance of its funds. It really was heaven sent. Rosemary could not wait to let the Trustees know but first she telephoned Dennis to put his mind at rest and then rushed to the bank in her lunch hour to put in the cheque.

'The Channel Four Documentary on the charity proved a huge success and became the beginning of an ongoing love affair between the charity and the media. Nina excelled in front of a camera and the dogs loved it. They not only loved playing to the camera but also to a live audience, as the charity was soon to discover.

'Smith's Charity, one of the Charitable Trusts to which Rosemary had written for funding responded positively and sent Virginia Graham down to assess the charity's suitability for funding. Rosemary and Nina met her at Kingsey House and the meeting seemed to go well. Unfortunately someone in the charity world happened to meet Virginia and expressed regret that Nina would shortly have to leave as her work permit would not be extended. Rosemary was unaware of this and it was like a bombshell when Virginia rang Rosemary to complain with some irritation and indignation that she had not been told about Nina's work permit problems as this obviously affected any decision her Trust might make on the funding application. Rosemary

50

apologised for not telling her and admitted that had she done so, she knew the chances of her application succeeding were zero. She went on to explain that on the basis that she was prepared to fight tooth and nail for Nina's right to stay in England permanently and that no decision had yet been made on that, she felt it prudent and in the charity's interest not to mention it. She also admitted that should Nina be deported and the charity had to close, then of course she would refund any money Smith's Charity might have given her. She gave her word on that. Virginia graciously accepted her argument and agreed to put the application before the Trust. To say Rosemary was relieved and delighted was perhaps an understatement!

'Not long after that, Rosemary was busy at work one morning when her telephone rang. It was David Carrick ringing to tell her that he had just heard from the MP to say that he had done everything he possibly could but the Home Office had decided to turn down Nina's application. He said that the MP could understand the reasons for that decision but was nonetheless very sorry. Rosemary was incandescent. She could not lose this fight. What a nightmare! She asked for the MP's telephone number at the House, which David gave her, and she rang him. He was very apologetic and said that he had the letter in front of him explaining the reasons for rejection but that it had not been sent yet. It was to be sent out that evening and once sent it would be extremely difficult to fight. He also explained that it would be helpful if she elicited the support of the Minister for the Disabled, who was William Hague at the time. At least Rosemary had a few hours to work with and asked for the letter to be faxed to her immediately. This was done. As she read it she knew she could ride a coach and horses through the arguments. Her computer at work did not have any word processing facilities, only spreadsheets, so she dashed in to her boss, explained the urgency of the situation and he agreed she should go home to write the letter to William Hague, which she did. She returned to the office and faxed the letter through. She also managed to obtain the direct telephone number of the top brass at the Home Office and then rang Lord Harewood and various other influential people pleading with them to contact the Home Office that day to stop this letter going out. As a result the letter was not sent and another reprieve was won.

'By this time Nina's expertise in dog behaviour and motivational training was rated so highly that she was considered one of the leading experts in the field. She was invited to address the British Small Animal Veterinary Association conference study on puppy assessment and she was also asked to give a presentation to the Geneva AFIRAC Conference, an international conference on human/animal interactions. Her expertise was being recognised across the world. The charity could not afford to lose her. Rosemary contacted the barrister working on Nina's behalf and discussed the whole situation with him. With his help Nina was eventually granted permanent residency. Rosemary was delighted to be able to ring Smith's Charity to tell them and to thank them for having faith in the charity.

'CPI received £20,000 from Smith's Charity to fund the appointment of a General Manager with an option to continue the funding for a second year. This provided a huge step forward. The charity had to move out of Kingsey House as it had only been taken on a short-term lease and David Carrick found premises in Havant, called Homewell House, the same building in which the MP worked. CPI took one room for the administrative staff. Ian Howard-Harwood was appointed General Manager in January 1995 and was ably supported by Jean MacKenzie, an administrative volunteer, who had been supporting the charity from the outset. Eventually a second room was taken for Nina.

'Due to the lack of funding and the difficulties over Nina's work permit the charity had not taken any more puppies into training. All efforts had been concentrated on getting the first three graduated. Money was now beginning to come in and it was agreed that more puppies could be purchased, so Nina was busy selecting the 'B' team. In the spring of 1995 Bracken, Bridie, Bertie, Basil, Badar and Biggles arrived. Heather Caird was appointed in June that year as an Assistant Trainer and from then on puppies have been brought in trained and graduated on a regular basis. During the financial year of 1995 over £100,000 was raised, which resulted in a surplus of £53,000. Most of the money donated was coming from charitable trusts. In the spring of 1995 Isobel Michael joined the Keith Davison firm and was given CPI as one of her projects. She suggested that an event be held to raise the profile of the charity and on 26th July 1995, CPI held their first demonstration aimed primarily at trusts, companies and influential people. This was a small affair held at Easthampstead Park Conference Centre near Wokingham. Isobel had, however, carefully researched the guest list.

'Nina put on a demonstration of the dogs' skills and they responded brilliantly. She really was an expert. One of the recipients talked about her life and how it had changed since the dog joined her and Rosemary talked about the charity and need for funds. At the end of that day over £60,000 was pledged and eventually received. Sky TV and local radio covered the event. The following year Isobel suggested that a much bigger event should be considered and in May 1996 another demonstration was put on at the Honourable Artillery Company in City Road, London, which was generously funded by the Libb Dupton Charitable Trust. That event produced nearly £100,000 and from it CPI made many valuable contacts who were to help the charity develop in the coming years.

'The scene was now set for the charity to develop. Administrative staff and training staff were taken on and the trainers moved to new premises in Steep Marsh near Petersfield in 1996.'

The charity is still flourishing today and has now realised Anne Conway's dream of having everything under one roof – dogs, residential training and offices in Heyshott near Midhurst. The possibility that the two similar charities should join together was discussed more than once. In September 2000, I was instructed by Dogs for the Disabled's Trustees to write to Rosemary Smith at Canine Partners for Independence asking that Trustees from the two charities should meet at the Wokingham guide dog centre. These and previous meetings always resulted in each group wanting to continue their independence in the way they had started. In recent years the Chairman and the Chief Executive of the two organisations have met annually to allow for cooperation and avoidance of conflicts.

Chapter 4

Dogs for the Disabled's early financial difficulties

Early successes with dogs began to show Frances' vision was possible. Dogs for the Disabled needed more money to continue its early start in producing a considerable number of assistance dogs, but the charity would grow slowly with difficulties. Compared with the problems that had faced its sister charity, Canine Partners, Dogs for the Disabled had fewer problems in training dogs in the first ten years, but the Trustees were faced with the need to bring in more money to run the charity. At times the problem seemed almost insurmountable, but a regular flow of income was necessary if the charity was to grow. The development of the use of assistance dogs through the charity founded by Frances Hay will be described in the next chapters.

Small individual donations to Dogs for the Disabled came in from people who had heard about these dogs; one or two legacy sums came in, often from people who appeared to have no connection with the charity. The name 'Dogs for the Disabled' did help to bring in support, and Trustee Ian Burr then suggested we paid to be listed in the publication used by solicitors and others when advising on suitable charities to include in wills. It was realised that it might take five to ten years before there was a steady flow of money from this source, but no one dreamt that twenty years later this would provide almost half the cost of running a much large charity providing dogs.

Finding the money to employ staff to train dogs was difficult in the early days, possibly because of the relationship developing with the well-established guide dog charity, there was a feeling that Dogs for the Disabled was then less in need of donations. After Frances died in 1990, one person's driving force was replaced by a group of Trustees who were committed to a greater or lesser extent to furthering the founder's ideas. The locations and setting for Dogs for the Disabled's work did not attract new support from the wealthy, nor get the attention of the main charitable trusts based in London and southern England. Fundraising in the Midlands continued to be the limiting factor in developing the charity, until eventually a major commercial supporter was found. Kenilworth, where Frances lived until her death, was a quiet residential town closely linked to the industrial Midlands for employment. Frances lived on the southern edge of the Coventry Green Belt countryside in an area only known for its ruined castle and its market gardens; 'Kenilworth' tomatoes were grown in nearby glasshouses in the sheltered warm valley and sold locally. It had much the appearance of a quiet Warwickshire market town where little had happened since Queen Elizabeth I's visit to the castle centuries earlier. Even the clock tower in the town centre remained unrepaired from a stray bomb dropped on Kenilworth in the 1940s which had landed at the central road junction.

Those who had come to see the charity found Frances' house on a corner, appropriately named Lower Ladyes Hill. The house, built on a slope, had necessitated Frances walking from her front door to reach her parked car, up a difficult slope. This may well have been where she had the idea of putting her dog on a tight lead to help her negotiate this slope to get to her vehicle. She not only kept her own two dogs in this terrace house but would take into her home 'dog prospects' for assessment, even though the house had only a small back yard.

A field opposite Frances' house was used to exercise dogs; it formed part of the Spring country estate, the home of a wealthy spinster, Miss Helen Martin, who bred white Standard Poodles. Following the owner's death, the estate was sold up, but Dogs for the Disabled was only very much later able to benefit from an anonymous trust fund set up in Miss Martin's memory. It had been my sad task to euthanase all the Poodles under the terms of Miss Martin's last will and testament; she did not want her dogs to be confined in kennels since they had always enjoyed the freedom of exercise in the extensive grounds around the house and farm.

The accommodation at Kenilworth was cramped; the underground basement of Frances' house was the original office for the charity. With extra secretarial help needing more space, the office was moved upstairs to a better-lit room on the first floor, next to Frances' bedroom. It may have been homely, but my impression after my first visit was that this charity was unlikely either to succeed or to survive long. Visitors were received in the front lounge of her house and were disappointed not to be able to be shown round any dogs in kennels.

At first, training was done from the homes in private houses, ideal in many ways for dogs that were intended to live in the homes of people with disabilities. With the major input from Jenny Cotton in Coventry, Frances trained the first dog, Rani, a bold German Shepherd, in this way. The first client, Mrs Gladys Rainbow, was a diabetic who had lost both her legs by amputation and then. as a result of a scald from hot coffee spilt on her lap, was unable to have artificial limbs fitted. After Rani had completed her training and been assessed by Frances as being of a suitable standard, a press launch for Rani with her new owner was held in Kenilworth's De Montfort hotel in spring 1988. A notice in the Dog World weekly newspaper reported that Gladys Rainbow, who used to show Poodles, had been given Rani to help her mobility. The launch in the hotel was attended by the Mayoress of Kenilworth and also invited were some of Frances' friends and a few local supporters. Invitations to the launch party were sent to other disability and dog charities; it brought along David Wilson from the Leamington GDBA, which was to have longer benefits than was realised at the time. The media were represented by one reporter from the local newspaper, the Kenilworth News. After Rani had been qualified with Gladys, the partnership never appeared in public again, but worked satisfactorily in Gladys' new home near Rugby.

Offers for help usually came from people wanting to give a dog to the charity, most dogs being unsuitable for training, since it was thought that they were just intended to act as companions for people in wheelchairs. There were no examples of dogs in kennels to demonstrate to visitors the type of dog required to perform the variety of skilled tasks.

Those early dogs selected for training were housed in supporters' homes in Coventry, Caroline Fraser, the second trainer, who later replaced Jenny Cotton, was given a free hand to find dogs and individually train them for the clients who had applied to the charity. Frances interviewed disabled clients on the telephone and later a three-page questionnaire was devised by the Trustees which allowed a better assessment of the needs and suitability of people to match with dogs. Prospective clients and dogs were found on a word of mouth basis. There were the radio interviews with Frances and later a memorable Blue Peter TV appearance that helped to spread the word about dogs working as 'assistants' to adults and children with disabilities.

In August 1988, the second assistance dog trained, Poppy, was given to Amanda Knapp, who had come from London for one week's residential training at Kenilworth. Caroline Fraser had trained the small 'rescued' Collie-cross bitch to work with a wheelchair user. With a dog like Poppy that would be working in London, there were new opportunities for publicity and to be able to show what an assistance dog was capable of. Until then, people in Great Britain only knew of the guide dogs used on the streets by blind people, and the long process of familiarisation with other dogs trained to assist in disabilities had begun.

Amanda in her wheelchair was the first person to ask her dog to retrieve the post once it came through the letterbox. When I visited her in her Kensington semi-basement flat, I was impressed that here was a dog doing an everyday task that had been previously impossible for a person in a chair to do. She had been unable to reach down and pick up a bundle of letters, a dropped pen or the TV remote control, but now all things previously inaccessible were quickly retrieved by Poppy at home.

Such simple tasks for a dog were later used in fundraising publicity, but it was not always easy to show how such a dog in the home could improve everyday existence for a person with specific disabilities. A scheme was set up where the supporters of the Dogs for the Disabled charity were invited to join on a membership basis as 'The Friends'; a small subscription gave them an embossed key ring and a newsletter which would be mailed to them.

In September 1988, the first promotional display for the charity was an exhibit at the veterinary nurses' congress at Stoneleigh, Warwickshire. I had a Leamington client from whom I borrowed a commercial poster advertising a girl with a Wella hairstyle for the exhibit. We had no display stands or promotional material. The improvised display stand created immediate interest amongst the veterinary nurses, since the model wore a dress similar to a nurse's uniform and she had a striking new hairstyle. The slogan attached to the poster stated that no other organisation had yet trained disability assistance dogs in the UK.

Leaflets were taken away by conference visitors and it brought in 45 new people as 'Friends', donating £3 each. The display was an opportunity to reach out to the veterinary practices, who would then receive a newsletter twice a year. The Trustees were looking for a corporate sponsor too amongst pet food manufacturers, but that only came much later. In 1988 the first of many newsletters was produced as a two-and-a-half page duplicated sheet, with the help of a Kenilworth publisher, who was one of Frances' supporters.

The Trustees of Dogs for the Disabled met monthly and they decided that instead of being a small charity in a small Midlands town, we should look for publicity in large cities, Birmingham and London being obvious targets. Christopher Timothy, the actor, who had appeared in the popular TV series built around the fictional vet James Herriot, was contacted by Frances and he willingly gave the new charity his support.

Amanda, with Poppy, organised a launch for the charity in London at the Tara Kensington Hotel in December 1988. Poppy, who had been trained with her in Coventry, was working well in London. A low budget party was set up by Amanda and the third dog to be assistance trained, Ben with Gina, would be ready to attend the launch party. The actor's presence at the hotel was helpful and he spoke favourably about the dogs and charged no fee.

At the hotel, Amanda Knapp with Poppy had spoken first to the small audience in the hotel room. Next Christopher Timothy said a few kind words, followed by Gina Geary, a severely disabled 23-year-old with spinal muscular atrophy. She spoke from her wheelchair with obvious passion. She had only come home from Coventry 10 days earlier with her new dog Ben. Gina was living in London, in a ground floor flat in Putney: she told how she had been dependant on 'carers' who sometimes had never arrived to help her. She spoke with great feeling about what having a dog had already done for her life. The dog was beside her 24 hours a day and she was no longer reliant on the people sent by Social Services. Her short talk, given with a convincing intensity, reminded me of Kerry Knaus, whom I had met in the States, at a similar age of 19, who had done so much to boost the appeal of Canine Companions for Independence when Bonita Bergin started training dogs in the USA.

Gina later wrote: 'People used to stare at me so I used to avert my face, but now I have Ben I can meet their eyes and they smile because they are looking at a beautiful dog, and we have a topic we can speak about without embarrassment. I find with Ben a rapport which is hard to establish with another human. I can confide in him without becoming vulnerable. He gives me independence which I could not achieve in any other way'.

Gina's dog Ben was an unwanted German Shepherd which suffered from a pancreatic deficiency. The digestive disorder needed special dietary care and Gina had the time to look after his needs to go outside frequently. I had first explained Ben's health problem to Gina when she came to Coventry for an assistance dog. She had stayed for the training in a disabled students' hostel, near to her trainer Caroline. The College was quiet, since it was not in term time, and during the fortnight's training course with Ben, Frances was supervising her too with frequent visits.

At the end of the second week, I visited Gina one evening in her student room in Coventry to make a qualifying health check on Ben before she went home. Later, as I had family living near Putney, I was able to visit Gina at home several times in London for aftercare support. Gina's shining personality with Ben, who accompanied her faithfully beside her wheelchair, made an excellent impression. She had spoken with a clear voice at the Tara Hotel about Ben as a 'rescued' dog. The dog's bowel disorder came to the attention of the American company Hills, who were able to offer a supply of special pancreatic diet food for Ben. The offer initially involved delivering their food to her flat free but for just six months. Gina wrote: 'Ben is extending my life in so many ways, pushing me into looking at the possible fulfilment of what were only dreams before'.

Gina's own health eventually deteriorated, but she had been able to visit Scotland as her first real holiday. In 1992, she moved away from South London to live in Scotland and was appointed Honorary Scottish Representative of Dogs for the Disabled. Next she moved to the East Midlands with a partner. They seemed happy together with Ben, but she lost many of her benefit payments. Since she was no longer living alone she had less of the living support money received before whilst in London.

When I went to see her again, she and her male partner seemed near destitute, not being able to buy petrol for their van. She went into a care facility for spinal disorders and Ben was retired to live with a friend, the end of a wonderful and supporting relationship.

The Tara Hotel event seemed helpful in promoting assistance dogs, but it did not produce the immediate national publicity Dogs for the Disabled had hoped for. At least there were no losses, as happened after Canine Partners' launch events in London later. The costs of the Tara Hotel refreshments were covered by visitors' donations, and there was no charge for the room. Unfortunately, as we had no public relations organisation to promote the event, no press or TV attended despite the many invitations to the media sent out by Frances.

Although the event had seemed low key with little publicity, there was a five-minute TV slot on the local channel 'London Plus', the first time the charity had access to the media. Amanda and Poppy were invited to appear and they were interviewed in December 1988. Later that year, an invitation came from BBC's Blue Peter children's show, which led to the appearance on January 9th 1989 of Amanda Knapp and her dog Poppy, together with Frances Hay.

The disappointing attendance at the hotel launch was now beginning to show that there were longer-term publicity benefits. The offer of free food for Ben also resulted in a promising offer of further support by Hills. The American-based company had quite recently come to market their dog foods in England, but needed to be known for producing specialist dog foods. They sold their 'Prescription Diets' exclusively to veterinary practices. Hills had a strong veterinary background in the States; they offered exclusive sales to veterinary surgeons who advised the food's use for dogs. The company had the vision to see that these trained assistance dogs would make ideal subjects to demonstrate how special diets could help to overcome any stresses in their work. Ross Tiffin for the Hill's Company said he hoped they would extend this support if the charity continued to grow.

In March 1989, it was arranged that Gina and Ben should appear at the World Small Animal Veterinary Congress to be held later that year in a Harrogate hotel. The congress meeting lasted several days and was attended by many delegates from the United Kingdom and from overseas. Gina made an impact there and further financial support followed from Hills, who were actively promoting their range of prescription diets to veterinary practices in this country and later in Europe. Ben had been on view at the WSAVA Harrogate Conference. When he had first arrived in Coventry he had been a thin German Shepherd with digestive difficulties. A year later he thrived on the new free diet food: he showed an immediate benefit, with a thicker coat and a less 'tucked up' abdomen.

Gina had been living alone, solely on state benefits, in her London flat, and the cost of feeding her new dog would have made life difficult for the two of them but for this new arrangement. The introduction of the Disability Living Allowance in 1988 had taken people out of residential care and the freedom to organise their own lives. It established for Gina the right to live in greater freedom, and the assistance dog movement became part of a greater individual freedom. Gina was a good example of the independent living that allowed an owner to enjoy her dog. Access rights made buildings and social events easier for Gina and Ben to reach in a wheelchair.

Hills were satisfied with the publicity and continued their support, and next they supplied help by the free use of a PR agent, Patric Judge. He worked for the firm KP & Co and would write press releases to publicise Dogs for the Disabled. He helped the charity to design a logo and provided other publicity material, such as window stickers, which was distributed to places where dogs had previously been denied access. Disabled people with their special needs needed to enter cafés and food shops or use public transport, but the presence of a dog could mean they were turned away. Disability 'rights' were then not understood and this required interventions by the charity.

Patric came to many of the committee meetings and helped to further the charity's image, increase public awareness and advise on steps we could take to help the clients. Hills became a major supporter for Frances, but were never willing to provide cash for the training work. Several hundred collecting boxes were made and Hills' veterinary representatives were to distribute these boxes and place them in the many veterinary clinics where interest had been shown.

Collection boxes were also put into Warwickshire public houses. When I heard one Warwick pub had changed landlords, I called in with a replacement box and was told by the new man 'there is no room for that in my bar'. This was almost the only denial I ever met in going round the country talking about assistance dogs.

The veterinary support for assistance dogs was furthered by an endorsement by the British Small Animal Veterinary Association (BSAVA) which led to an arrangement for six-monthly veterinary health checks for dogs being established. The arrangement was similar to the scheme for guide dog biannual inspections. Health books were printed with a design similar to those used by the GDBA, and free booster vaccinations were arranged on an annual basis by BSAVA small animal vets. Clients were also issued with identity cards which carried the new Dogs for the Disabled logo of a client in a wheelchair with a dog beside it.

Frances had always been very good at making personal contacts to promote the charity, but few had led to new sources of regular income. On one occasion, in September 1989, she was asked to speak at a national conference held at Peterhouse College in Cambridge organised by UFAW (The Universities Federation for Animal Welfare) on 'training working dogs'. Her contribution was fairly disjointed: she said the dogs would 'not only give physical help but also provide people with important psychological aspects of love and affection, companionship, sense of security and, above all, a feeling of independence and confidence'.

The information she gave about her training methods was unfortunately passed over, with so many other more professional speakers making greater impact. Her health was already beginning to fail and although she was offered an overnight room in the College, she decided to drive home with her two dogs the same evening. The return journey to Kenilworth should have taken two and a half hours, but in fact it took her a lot longer, after she first got lost trying to leave the city and next set off in the wrong direction. She finally arrived home in Kenilworth at three in the morning, she told me. She was accompanied in the car by her two demonstration dogs, Misty and Kim, and she must have driven in circles taking many wrong turnings trying to return in the dark from Cambridge. The doctor ordered two weeks' complete rest and Doreen took on the task of banking the incoming donations, tending the garden, collecting shopping and various other duties.

Publicity was not easy to obtain, and sometimes external events worked against us. I was invited to speak about assistance dogs work at an animal welfare meeting held in November 1987 at Regents Park, London Zoo, and afterwards I gave an interview about the dogs to a reporter from The Times. Tragically, the same night at Kings Cross Underground, a fire caused the loss of many lives. Descriptions of these events took over the media and only the briefest of reports on assistance dogs appeared in the early newspaper editions the next day. All the national newspapers were taken over with photos of the fire and accounts of the victims of the accident where many lives had been lost.

Thinking that Birmingham, closer to hand, would be a better place to get the media's attention, a new publicity strategy was next tried. With Frances' health problems it was decided that she needed more professional help and she invited an old acquaintance of hers, Mike Hartley, to join her with charity promotion work. He had contacts with the BBC and had previously interviewed Frances on the radio. The audiotape shows that he had interviewed her about the problems of artificial legs, which were dealt with in a fairly light hearted manner. In answering questions from callers she did say that 20 years after her operation she was still getting phantom pain in the leg stump. Mike, after his unofficial recruitment by Frances, was asked to meet the Trustee committee in September 1990. Mike was very plausible with TV experience and had his own film company he said, so he was engaged as a paid consultant and part-time worker to help with organisation. There was the promise that his own firm, Friss Films, would make a promotional video for the charity. The bargain price for it was negotiated by the dog food manufacturer, but unfortunately nothing was ever delivered. He was given a free hand by Frances and the one action he will be remembered for was using his Birmingham TV connections to get one of the assistance dogs on a peak time viewing national show. Saturday Night Live was a very popular programme produced by Granada in their Birmingham studio; it went out every week on all UK channels.

In retrospect, I have a fair idea of how this was arranged or 'set up' by Mike Hartley. He had previously been a disc jockey on a late night show with the BBC Birmingham at the time of 'song plugging'. After that, he was very reluctant for his name to appear or be used later for this TV event. A health campaign against the high sugar content of many foods was in the news, as there is again today. The promotion in the late 1980s was a health drive initiative, to reduce the sugar contents of food. Tate & Lyle, one of the principle sugar manufacturers, became a target, and they were induced to come on the Saturday night show to defend their profit making with their sugar cane plantations overseas.

This rather unexpectedly provided Mike Hartley with an angle to introduce a dog into the TV show. Tally was a Golden Retriever trained by Dogs for the Disabled. She had been obtained from the GDBA and on qualifying Tally had gone out to be with an elderly ex-serviceman, Len, a double amputee using a wheelchair. He lived on his own in sheltered accommodation at Chelmsley Wood, close to Birmingham. In his hand-propelled wheelchair he got around and was well known in his locality. He was astonished when at first Tally would stop and sit at every kerb edge just as a dog for the blind would. Unfortunately, as well as Len being a heavy smoker (which at first made his dog cough, until this was pointed out to him), he was heavily built and his food habits were extended to 'Tally', who also became overweight within months of his receiving her in October 1989.

Unlike the dog's cough problem, on which he had cooperated when asked by opening the windows, this new problem of the dog's weight gain was not being controlled. Tally was suddenly removed from him by Mike Hartley for 'dieting'. Not unexpectedly, Len objected to losing the dog and spoke out in the local press about his dog being taken from him. He obtained some sympathy. Press enquiries were dealt with by saying it was done for the dog's health. but it did seem to many rather harsh for this to have been carried out with little warning.

After Tally had been away from Len for six weeks or so in kennels, Mike arranged for the now slimmer dog to be handed back to Len in full view of the TV cameras on the Granada TV Saturday night show. I agreed to go over to help Frances at this event and we were collected by a Granada limousine from her house, early on the Saturday evening. Mike, already at the studios and in charge, then decided Frances should not be the person to hand the dog over. She was promised she could sit in the front row of the audience with the understanding the cameras would pick her out. Tally was to be handed over to me, where we would renew our acquaintance, which was not difficult since I had known the dog from several previous occasions after treating her cough from the passive smoking problem.

Before the handover there had been a free drinks session at the bar laid on by Granada. I was wary of this but asked for a whisky to be kept under their bar for me until after the show. Those invited, including Frances and Len, were able to indulge freely with the alcohol as they wished. I was then led off to a private dressing room; Mike appeared with Tally on a lead and next I was placed behind a screen in the dark at the back of the studio. There was a lot of noise in the front, but having known Tally before, I reassured her by talking gently, as the noise from the other side of the screens was increasing and it was disturbing her.

I was then given the nudge by a prompter to walk the dog forward. Two doors were flung open and we were both in the full glare of studio lights with a crescendo of music. Apparently the plan had been that when Len saw his dog again he would burst into tears and the message that a slim dog was better than an obese one would not be lost on the audience, who had just had the dangers of excess sugar in foods explained.

The plan fell flat. Unfortunately Len, who had experienced much worse things as a World War II survivor, accepted his dog without a quiver or a tear! Alcohol had not altered his behaviour in the way TV producers must have found with others appearing on such shows, where violent emotional outbursts were encouraged. Frances sat bemused in the front row and on viewing the replays later only got the briefest of silent camera time. Somehow the show had not had the publicity impact intended, since the audience were more confused by the effect of sugar in their foods and the dog's presence seemed irrelevant.

Mike Hartley came up with more ideas. One of the two cars leased by Dogs for the Disabled was being kept at his home outside Birmingham rather than being available as a pool car for the trainers. His film seemed not to be progressing. Other expenses were claimed on the charity, but the expenditure he proposed was shooting up way ahead of our small income. Fortunately David Wilson from the GDBA had joined as a Trustee in December 1989, only a year before Frances tragically died. David had worked in the motor industry; he had a financial control background and alerted the other Trustees to the situation of Mike Hartley's expenditure and free use of a car that had been arranged with Frances. Frances' father, George, as one of the Trustees, was concerned too and afterwards told me of other irregularities that took place. To cover costs, which exceeded income, £5000 had to be taken from a small reserve at the bank which had been built up slowly to cover for outgoings and a halt put on all new expenditure or purchases.

A separate contract for Friss Films with Hills had been negotiated by Mike for £10,000, but no promotional film was ever produced.

There was a difficult financial situation which had to be controlled. At the final Trustees' meeting in December 1990, Frances attended as the Director General. It was proposed that she should be moved 'sideways' and given the title 'Founder and President of DFD'. One of the Trustees was medically qualified and it had become obvious that the founder was no longer able to be in effective control of the charity that she had started only a few years earlier.

Frances died in Selly Oak Hospital on December 22nd 1990, from acute liver failure. Her father and daughter were in the USA and she had driven herself to a hospital she knew and arranged for herself to be admitted.

On January 19th 1991 the Trustees held a meeting at the GDBA's Edmonscote Manor. Following Frances' death, arrangements had been made for her funeral and cremation at Oakleigh Wood earlier that day. I was celebrating my 60th birthday in Scarborough on the day Frances died. On arriving at the hotel, our group first had to go through a police check as there was a political conference that weekend. The hotel reception asked me to make a phone call to Florida. George told me of his daughter's death and he was adamant that Mike Hartley was to have no part in arranging the funeral, which must wait until his return as executor. I then had to contact Hartley and tell him his short-term contract had expired on December 23rd and apart from completing his film he would not be required again by the Trustees. He was informed that a new administrator was required for the charity.

At the meeting on January 9th, one of the items dealt with was a salary claim by Mike Hartley as well as the return of the loaned car. There was also a problem of the missing Butchers Tripe money, which was never solved. The funeral was reported in the local press, and I had written a tribute to Frances on January 11th which had been published in the weekly papers covering the dog world. It was not until

January 29th that an obituary, written by Neil Ewart, appeared in The Independent.

The charity moved its office to Edmonscote Manor on January 2nd and Doreen Cross agreed to continue as secretary there in temporary accommodation, assisted by Linda Crawley. The financial situation of the charity by the January 1991 was so serious that debts of £2000 could only be cleared when an unexpected legacy for a slightly larger amount arrived by the end of the month to restore the bank account. The Trustees were relieved by the arrival of this unexpected sum, as well as another small legacy, to feel that right was on their side in keeping the charity alive after these gifts arrived. There was only one dissenting Trustee. who wanted to wind up the business as there was such a small income flow. Fortunately for the future, he was outvoted and plans were made on how to keep the charity running. The solicitors to the F Hay estate asked for payment of £602 arrears of her wages, causing another unexpected demand. When the charity was registered in 1988, Frances as Director General was initially on £500 per annum token salary, which had been increased in 1990 to £1000 plus her expenses. The money was found for her estate. but new income was slow to arrive. Frances' house was required to be sold at once and the charity became temporarily homeless.

The Trustees set about putting the charity on a firmer footing. A regular income flow was urgently needed, sponsorship was discussed and ways of increasing the number of dogs trained became priorities. More dogs trained and out amongst the public would improve the charity's image. Despite an increasing public awareness, money was coming in only in small amounts: a donation of £250 from the Spastics Society was one, followed by £500 from the Kenilworth Round Table. Local firms such as Colan, with safety clothing, and Trust Pet Products helped with some of the running costs of dog training. Small sums were coming in on an irregular basis from many sources.

Early in December 1990, the first approach had been made to the

Director General of the GDBA for financial support for training by Dogs for the Disabled. It was not possible for the senior charity, established in the 1930s to help blind people, to give funds directly to another dog-based charity. It was thought possible for them to give help in other ways; trainers could be seconded to other types of dog work to enhance their dog training skills, and equipment could be loaned, together with advice on sources for suitable dog selection. The Dogs for the Disabled Trustees decided about this time that 'rescue' dogs were too uncertain in temperament to spend a lot of time on training only to find them unreliable as assistance dogs.

From the very beginning, Frances and her father were offering training for 'unwanted and abandoned dogs' and had used the slogan when appealing for money. Frances' father objected to no longer being able to use rescue dogs but he had to be overruled by those now preparing the dogs. He had used the 'unwanted and abandoned dogs' title when writing appeals for money.

Once Caroline Fraser retired, followed by her death after a sudden illness, no more rescue dogs were used. The new trainers from the GDBA were more accustomed to the larger breeds used as guide dogs. Lessons had been learnt by what one might expect from trying to arrange publicity from a single appearance of one of the assistance dogs. Appearing on the Blue Peter children's programme in 1989 had made only a small impact, although previously over many years a guide dog puppy had been brought in to the children's programme on a regular basis by Derek Freeman. Honey the Labrador developed an enormous following for many years, having made her first appearance on TV when seven weeks old and qualified as a guide dog for school teacher Elsie.

Derek, a bluff Yorkshireman, fitted the image of a countryman and dog trainer, and he had the confidence of Biddy Baxter, the programme producer, who gave him regular appearances on her show from 1964 onwards. Derek's book Barking up the Right Tree described many of the episodes of the TV programme he was called to join in. Guide dog puppies Honey, Cindy, Buttons and Goldie successively became many children's favourites and parents took notice of benefits of dogs with children. The TV dogs in the programme often became substitute dogs for children where pets could not be accommodated due to housing and other restrictions on keeping a pet at home. Unfortunately Dogs for the Disabled never achieved such popularity, but it was arranged that when in a litter of puppies was born to a GDBA Labrador bitch their development would be followed. One would need to be 'rejected' for training' on temperament, but it would be given to the assistance dog charity to train.

Once the link to the GDBA had been firmly established there were fewer difficulties in finding skilled dog trainers The supply of dogs was quite good and accommodation for staff and dogs was well above the standard in the dog industry. It was made clear from the first Letter of Arrangement drawn up between the two charities that there would be no direct cash input from the large and wealthy charity into the small 'starting from nothing' Dogs for the Disabled. Full-time staff could now be directly employed by the charity to help the two part-time secretaries of Frances Hay, Doreen and Linda.

A young lady who had recently been trained with an attractive Labrador, Elton, was chosen as a fundraiser who would provide a suitable image to follow the work of Frances Hay. Parry was to go out as a paid fundraiser; it was thought a young woman with an attentive yellow Labrador would provide an image for what the charity's work was about. Local fundraising events and a grant from the Percy Bilton charitable trust meant that could start her work in July 1991, a local girl who had suffered an injury whilst still at school, was quite mobile but had no transport available to get her out to events; the following year she was allocated the use of an ex-GDBA staff car. Fundraising was often erratic and unpredictable: a stall set up by the charity at the Festival of Bernese dog show at Stoneleigh Royal Showground raised just £36. A model of a wooden dog was donated by a Kenilworth toymaker and it was put on display with a collecting box, but income was poor. The Cubbington Brownies and the Leamington Women's Royal Naval Club were donors that helped to keep the charity alive, and more help came when the Leamington Lions' organisation purchased 18 sets of dog equipment for our future needs. In 1991 it was all welcome support, until eventually a major sponsor could be found. Larger donations came in too from the Lions club and the Leamington travel agents Lunn Poly with £1000 each.

A fundraising branch in Oswestry, with Sir Michael Leighton as chairman, had been set up through a personal contact and the appointment of the golfer Ian Woosnam as the President of the branch was warmly welcomed as an entry into the world of golf and potential fundraising by golf clubs. A cheque for £2000 for Dogs for the Disabled, together with a congratulatory message from Ian, was the first result. Later, other golf clubs raised money for Dogs for the Disabled too.

Two months later, Hills, the dog food manufacturer which had earlier given limited support, were again approached. In view of the new situation, with more dogs coming along, they agreed to contribute £10,000 towards the cost of an 'administrator'. Their support was welcome, since another leading food manufacturer had rejected our advances and they were assumed to be already supporting the other assistance dog charity.

A person to head the charity would be recruited with a salary of around £15,000 per annum. Adverts were placed in a national newspaper, as this was then felt a realistic sum to attract the right person. Hills, as sponsor, would deliver a free supply of dog food for all dogs trained and offered their own retained PR company to help with publicity. The sponsorship was a considerable step forward in establishing the charity nationally.

The death of Frances and her vision had made an impact on organisations that previously might have held back their support for a new and 'untried' dog charity. More help was soon to follow with training the dogs. Helen McCain came from Exeter to Leamington as the first of two trainers seconded from the guide dog organisation; she gave her committed involvement to assistance dogs to provide more professional training and dog selection. She had first been introduced to the work of the charity when she had accompanied George Cram to meet the client Ann Greenwood with Shep in Cornwall. In 1992 the Trustees decided to ask for another trainer to be loaned, on the basis that the charity was expanding and the job offered an opportunity for more GDBA specialist trainers to enlarge their skills working dogs with other disabilities. Of the first 18 trained dogs, eight came from guide dog training centres, so it was in their organisations' interests to be involved in aftercare visits to these dogs as well as in their training. The idea was helped with the first 'dual dog', a black Labrador, Susannah, which had been placed with a blind lady living in Cardiff. She had lost both of her legs and relied on a wheelchair to get her around in her sheltered housing courtyard. When visited she told me she was so pleased that now she had Susannah, as the dog would take her round the paved area and guide her to the homes of some of her disabled friends who lived nearby. Before Susannah came she could only sit indoors all day until someone came to take her out.

More practical help came when Neil Ewart from the guide dog breeding centre was appointed as unpaid training adviser. He attended all Trustee monthly meetings and with his experience had a tremendous influence on the selection of dogs and their use as assistance dogs. He was also involved with BBC's Blue Peter, and when he took five puppies to the studios in March 1991, he was able to predict from their temperament that one pup would 'not make it as a guide dog trainee' but could be eminently suitable as a dog for a disabled applicant.

Within three or four months of Frances' untimely death, the charity really seemed to be moving forward and support was coming from many unexpected directions. In 1992, two years after Frances Hay had died, the charity had progressed with the appointment of David Bennet as the first full-time Chief Executive. A new GDBA contract was made for Neil Ewart to act as Training Consultant one day a week, and with help by George Cram, a guide dog trainer at their Exeter Centre, it put Dogs for the Disabled on a firmer basis.

A demand for dogs in the South West of England grew due to publicity around the Blue Peter appearance of Shep. Early in 1992 a second trainer from GDBA volunteered to come to help with training, and Angela Pinder worked with Helen in late January. She was an ex-employee of GDBA but after an overseas break she had shown interest in coming back to training work, and she could live with GDBA staff at Tollgate House where the office and kennels were in use.

Just over a year later fundraising was improving with £42,000 funds available. The Percy Bilton charity was the first major donor and other sources were beginning to come through. After one Trustee meeting it was suggested that Frances Hay should receive a permanent and greater acknowledgment, and the portrait painter Roger Clark, working in the Cotswolds, was approached. A fee was negotiated, a few photos of her were provided and several months later all the Trustees travelled to the small village where the painting was viewed and approved in its final stages. On delivery it was hung in a prominent place at the offices of Dogs for the Disabled, and later it was hung in the Old Vicarage kennels at Ryton on Dunsmore. The fee for the portrait was paid out of charity funds on the basis of it being publicity material. Later we were informed that each Trustee should have made an equal contribution out of their own pocket to cover the cost, since it was not a charitable requirement. Years later the portrait mysteriously vanished from display on the wall and was said to have been stored in the cellars of the Old Vicarage, a property owned by the GDBA with parts leased to Dogs for the Disabled. When independence came with the National Lottery award that allowed the move to Banbury, the portrait could not been found. It was rumoured that like the Graham Sutherland portrait of Winston Churchill, our modest portrait had offended someone, and they had taken an axe to it in the cellars. In the last 25 years the whole 'disability revolution' has transformed society and lives, but regrettably some person was responsible for this unexplained act of destruction in the late 1990s of a pioneers' portrait.

Bonita Bergin came to the GDBA's Tollgate House to talk about her experiences developing Canine Companions for Independence as a charity in the USA. Her experiences were listened to closely and gave confidence to continue the expansion of Dogs for the Disabled. The five Trustees, the training staff and other invited supporters there were all inspired by what she had done in the USA. A proposal was made that we should ask her to give a boost to the charity by providing staff training and management for the British charity, but the overall cost of the training package was something the GDBA could not take on under the banner of staff development. The opportunity was lost for a 'leap forward' and it was reluctantly decided that the growth of Dogs for the Disabled would have to proceed slowly as money became available. Fundraising in a more organised and professional manner would have to be a priority.

Being based in the Midlands close to the GDBA centres, the charity was slow to make an impact in southern England, where there was greater wealth and many of the large trusts and the large companies were based. After organisational problems and the departure of the first male Chief Executive inside six months, a 'Training Manager' instead was chosen to be recruited to head the staff, as a person who had greater practical experience of working dogs. Soon after the appointment of Linda Hams, I well remember travelling to London with her as we had obtained an appointment with one of the 'big five' banks in the hope of endorsement and sponsorship. We were welcomed by a director of their charitable giving arm, and given coffee in pleasant surroundings where we presented our case. We came away with the promise that the Bank would pay for some display boards that we could take round with us to outdoor events. It was not the large sum we asked for, and this was the token level of support that we got from many applications to likely donors.

Other approaches were made, but money was not easy to find. We decided next to recruit a person to head the appeals and organise a more regular supply of income. It was at a time when the offices in a bungalow at Tollgate House were no longer available, since planning permission for the use of the rooms had been withdrawn.

The GDBA wanted to set out a firmer financial basis for their input into this 'sister charity' and it had been found by their governing council that in their constitution they could become a corporate trustee of local charities. This clause was probably introduced in the past to allow them to give money to charities dealing with the welfare of blind and partially-sighted people. It proved a wonderful opportunity for Dogs for the Disabled to benefit from a firm connection to the much larger and more financially-successful charity.

The Chairman wrote to the GDBA Board stating that the idea was welcomed, as it would allow DFD to operate individually; the memory of Frances Hay would be preserved. Fundraising by Dogs for the Disabled would be allowed to operate competitively and independently with GDBA there to underwrite, when needed, the supply and the training of dogs, etc (quote from Trustee minutes, April 22nd 1991). Even though only four of our Trustees were at this meeting, a strong case was made to follow this route. Discussion went on into the late evening and eventually all were convinced that this proposal by the GDBA would not be harmful and the risk of being swallowed up by a more powerful neighbour was not a threat to independent action.

Chapter 5

The unexpected death of Frances Hay and the years that followed

Dogs for the Disabled urgently needed more money to build on its early start in producing successfully-working assistance dogs. The charity had first started as a family group with a few friends, using Frances' house as a base. Following her unexpected death, the charity needed to move on, building up new connections and operating as a business with the much longed-for cash flow. The search for a corporate sponsor continued. The charity was too small and largely unproved in its work to attract a major backer, but financial support eventually came from unexpected sources that allowed for full independence with the move to Banbury.

Frances had been able to bring in volunteers who had experience of dog training and had worked in local dog clubs. She relied on her father, George Newns, to oversee the difficult financial side, since funds were few and far between; he also advised on who he thought could become suitable Trustees to get the charity registered with the

Charity Commission. Frances' daughter Deborah, too, was involved in exercising the dogs and was a great support to her mother.

Following Frances' death in December 1990, the next issue of the newsletter was hurried out, devoted to 'Frances Hay's Great Legacy' with numerous tributes to her work. A quote from the mother of a child with spina bifida who had been given a dog was printed as a mark of respect:

'He's virtually indispensable. He picks up everything my daughter drops, which is particularly useful because of her spinal jacket. At night, if there's an emergency, he barks to wake me up. He's learnt to 'speak' so that he can tell me when she needs me.'

The work an assistant dog could do was beginning to be recognised by the public, and plans had to be drawn up to continue the work. First priority was to find a new training base away from Frances' home. A vacant Portakabin had been found at the Leamington GDBA Centre and was offered for use as temporary offices early in 1991. Frances' house was cleared within weeks of her death. A small amount of equipment such as a donated manual typewriter and a filing cabinet were removed from the Lower Ladyes Hill house, which needed to be emptied quickly for selling. Doreen and Lynda, as part-time secretaries for Frances, were able to move into a new light and airy office at the GDBA Leamington centre.

Interest was now taken by trainers of guide dogs at the centre and a mutual respect developed. Neil Ewart and Mike Cembrovicz, employed by the GDBA, were particularly supportive in those first early months. In the previous year, some of the trainers' meetings had been held at the GDBA Breeding Centre kennels at Tollgate House. The move of the Dogs for the Disabled office to a guide dog centre did not cause any great difficulties other than all phone calls and enquiries to Dogs for the Disabled charity having to go through the GDBA manual switchboard.

In April 1991, the Trustees invited the GDBA organisation to become more closely involved and appoint persons to the Dogs for the Disabled board. The 'corporate Trustee' was appointed to allow GDBA to have a direct involvement in the management but without overall control. In August 1991, the Charity Commissioners stated there was no objection to the Association acting as a corporate Trustee for Dogs for the Disabled. Following Frances' death, the number of Trustees was increased to nine, allowing a wider range of skills to be brought in. The financial situation was improving. £16,695 had been received from The Percy Bilton Trust during the year, an increase from the £5,565 received grant in the previous year. A legacy for £21,000 had also been received, so £40,000 could be put into a reserve fund. David Wilson, as a newer Trustee who was a GDBA employee, suggested we should have a client with a working dog employed on a full time basis, for publicity. It would increase the paid staff and she would be helped by the two part-time secretaries already working from the Portakabin. There was a need to expand dog the training too, as the list of applicants for dogs was at 200 and increasing. There was only one full-time trainer seconded from the GDBA and Caroline Fraser as the part- time trainer, who was working from her home in Coventry. Caroline did not drive, so this limited her activities, especially when after-care visits were needed. Sheba, a German Shepherd cross, was the last dog of nine she trained for the charity.

A request was made for another trainer who could be seconded by the GDBA and for the dogs to be based and trained at GDBA's Tollgate House, just outside Leamington. The Tollgate kennels were run by Derek Freeman to breed puppies for the GDBA. He loved anything to do with dogs and the new arrangement to have a new sort of training taking place there seemed very amicable.

The house and grounds, purchased some years earlier by the GDBA, was a substantial country house with fields around, previously used by a Mr Brooks for growing mushrooms to go into meat pies. It was listed as an agricultural site with a turkey farm adjacent. In the 1960s the GDBA had started a breeding scheme. When it expanded and they needed a new site in the country, kennels were built at Tollgate for the GDBA dog breeding centre and there was spare capacity for additional dog activities. The composition of the board of Trustees of Dogs for the Disabled was realigned, consisting of five Trustees from GDBA and four who were independent of the larger charity; there was no point of contention as it was arranged in the spirit of a developing partnership.

Doreen and Linda continued as secretarial staff in the Portakabin, with the first computer word processor, Linda also moving to Tollgate later. The £750 received from Telethon Central TV's show where Len and Tally had appeared, was allocated for the purchase of the first computer connected for use in the Portakabin office. The purchase and setting up was done by a young Leamington man who had just received a grant from the Princes Trust to set up his own business, helping him to establish himself as well. The temporary office Portakabin was available as the charity's single office until another move became necessary in February 1992. The staff in the GDBA Training Department, who had been based in Derek Freeman's staff bungalow, were relocated to their head office at Wokingham, which allowed our charity's office to move into the vacant bungalow at GDBA's Tollgate site. Close to the kennels, the new building, on Green Belt land, had planning permission as accommodation for the dog breeding manager.

After Derek Freeman moved away with a growing family, the larger rooms in the vacant bungalow were used as a temporary office. The GDBA agreed that two office rooms could be leased to Dogs for the Disabled, as well as the use of six kennels for dogs in an adjacent kennel block. It was quite easy for a bedroom in the bungalow to be adapted to provide accommodation for a disabled person who might come in for residential training by Dogs for the Disabled with a dog. The room was furnished and shown to visitors but was never used for a training class person, since a nearby motel was available with better support.

As the charity grew, a new appointment to improve the administration of the charity was authorised by the Trustees as more money became available; David Bennet came from the Shaw Trust charity to fill a new Chief Executive post. The second trainer for the dogs in kennels became possible when Angela came up from the Exeter GDBA Centre to work beside Helen McCain, who had moved into Tollgate House to live.

We were already looking to the future; the Trustee minutes of 1992 show that I prepared a memorandum on the future of Dogs for the Disabled. Trustee Ian Burr was asking then for some research into the benefits of dogs to disabled people and of the types of disabilities where the greatest benefit could be expected. It was not clear who would fund research. Trustee David Wilson said Pedigree Petfoods was sponsoring the other assistance dog charity, ADDP (Assistance Dogs for the Disabled People) for three years. Dogs for the Disabled's food supplier, Hills did not offer further funding; it was many years before any research was possible. Fortunately Hills still allowed Patric Judge of the publicity agents KP & Co to continued to write press releases.

The training of more assistance dogs to keep up with the increasing waiting list became the next priority. In order to learn more, the GDBA sponsored two of their staff, Helen McCain and Paul Master, to travel to the USA to attend one of Bonita Bergin's Service Dogs Seminars. The GDBA had offered continuing support to Dogs for the Disabled for one to five years, saying it was easier to provide dog trainers to work at Dogs for the Disabled as their career development, rather than direct payments or anything else not connected to blindness. Helen was accordingly next invited to attend a six-week training course at the Bonita Bergin College in California at a cost of £1500 plus travel & accommodation costs, all of which was paid for by the GDBA. It was about this time that 'clicker' training of dogs came into use as the method of 'positive reinforcement' used in the training routine; food rewards and praise, both verbal and patting, were continued as well.

Income in 1991 was slowly improving, with £60,000 in the first seven months, which included a £20,000 legacy. Money was beginning to arrive from new sources as the work of assistance dogs became better known. A cheque from the Royal Veterinary Colleges Students' Union for £850 was received as the proceeds of the Bicentenary Ball. Colin Plum, a GDBA staff member and valued supporter, proposed setting up a local fundraising branch in Cubbington with Debby Parry, the new fundraiser's help, on 10th September 1991. With the GDBA's knowledge of possible conflict in fundraising, Cubbington, as a Leamington suburb, was chosen rather than Warwick. There was an understanding that Dogs for the Disabled would not open support groups at places in competition with existing GDBA branches. There was already an active GDBA branch in Leamington run by Muriel Evans.

In September that year, I was asked to go to Cheshire to speak to the newly-formed Dogs for the Disabled Wirral branch, at the invitation of Mrs Marion Garrett. The Wirral Branch had raised £1200, as there was already a successful Dogs for the Disabled partnership working there and an active supporters' group. I drove up after work, arriving at 8 pm to give my talk to find a room filled with enthusiastic supporters. I returned home on the same Monday evening; I do not recall that I even charged any travel expenses, since I was driving my veterinary practice work car.

A week later, a letter came from Julie Hindle wanting to start training assistance dogs in Cheshire. It would have been a good opportunity to expand more quickly, but the request was rejected by the enlarged board of Trustees as it was felt it would be impossible to control the training standards of the dogs. There was an air of caution, as the assistance dog idea seemed to be capturing more public interest in what dogs might be able to do. The members appointed by the GDBA on the board wanted our charity to grow organically and not take unnecessary risks.

George Newns had submitted a paper to the other Trustees on continuing to use 'rescue' dogs in our publicity: Frances' father, as a founder Trustee, asked that the use of 'abandoned' dogs for training should again be discussed. Caroline Fraser told the meeting that in the past four years she had trained seven rescue dogs. There were only a few problems found, of a rescue dog growling at children and a rescue German shepherd becoming too protective of its home. Both events were temporary phases and had been dealt with, she said. George Newns felt embarrassed, since administrators of the Douglas Trust had donated money on the basis that some rescue dogs would be used in training. Although George had some successes, he said that Bonita Bergin, after her visit, would not use the emotional appeal of rescue dogs for fundraising purposes but rely on projecting the professionalism, as with her USA organisation.

Carolyn Fraser was instructed to take in, on approval only, a 'rescued' dog that the training consultant Neil Ewart had first seen and assessed. Unfortunately she did not have the capability of training this type of dog, and with her developing health problem she retired from her work for Dogs for the Disabled before succumbing to her final illness. Carolyn and her daughter Fay were pioneers of Frances' wish to help people with disabilities; they have largely been forgotten, except by clients such as Ann Greenwood, whose first dog she had trained.

George Newns approached Pedigree Petfoods for sponsorship, but the firm declined. Their reply from Michael Jenkins stated, 'It makes eminent sense to me that in order to maximise awareness and future growth, ADDP and DFD should consider a merger, but I cannot meddle in internal politics'. The Trustees had decided that in view of the new relationship with GDBA, a merger with ADDP was a non-starter and fundraising would continue without mentioning using abandoned dogs. The recycled part-trained guide dogs were being used by Dogs for the Disabled but could not be classified as unwanted rescue dogs. There were benefits for both the two cooperating charities. Labradors and Retrievers trained by the GDBA for many months were not wasted if they were then found temperamentally unsuited to working in traffic guiding blind persons.

Dogs for the Disabled immediately gained by receiving dogs that had already undergone extensive training that could be converted to retrieve and give support to people with disabilities other than visual impairment. Offers of more dogs for use by Dogs for the Disabled came in from the four main GDBA training centres, but the strongest link was now being made with their centre at Exeter. George Cram and Carolyn Bull were both working from Exeter training disability dogs and making aftercare visits in the West Country.

Bonita Bergin continued her interest in Dogs for the Disabled and came to visit the Tollgate House GDBA breeding centre and to inspect the Dogs for the Disabled arrangements. Bonita had come over again from California after being invited to speak at a one-day seminar organised at the Royal Veterinary College Campus, and the meeting was attended by GDBA staff as well as by the London College's veterinary students. Further cooperation seemed possible with her USA assistance dog organisation Canine Companions for Independence (CPI). After her visit on Sept 12th 1991, Bonita wrote to GDBA's David Wilson (as one of our Trustees) with a plan for instructing 'service training' of dogs at each of the seven GDBA centres. It was a bold plan to allow rapid expansion of training dogs for all disabilities. The proposal was a plan estimated to cost $672,000. It included her travel, accommodation and consulting fees to be completed by the 'fall' of 1992 with seven more dogs she would have trained for Dogs for the Disabled. She had also advised breeding our own dogs in future, rather than relying on gifted and purchased puppies. The cost was larger than the GDBA were prepared to underwrite and it was feared that the blind communities and users of guide dogs, who had been the charity's main beneficiaries since 1932, would not countenance such a change in a new direction.

The seminar also resulted in more cooperation with the College in London, after a video was made there by Dr Jenny Poland's audio-visual unit about the four types of assistance animals. Plans for European satellite TV broadcasts funded by British Telephones were made by Dr Poland using her contacts through the audio-visual unit. Two sessions in a Europe educational slot were set up by Barcud North Wales studios. Further funding from European sources did not come in to allow the project to continue, but the publicity obtained was of value for future developments.

Dr June McNicolas from Warwick University came with me to one of the TV studio discussions, which helped to further the connection that led to the first research project with Warwick in 1994. The cooperation was to be a crucial factor later in obtaining funding from the National Lottery, who asked to see any research results.

By 1992 as well as having David Bennet appointed as Chief Executive, the GDBA offered a contract for the experienced Neil Ewart to act as our Training Consultant one day a week, helped by George Cram, a senior guide dog trainer based at their Exeter centre. A demand for dogs in the South West of England grew due to continuing publicity for Ann Greenwood's dog Shep.

Early in 1992 a second trainer from GDBA volunteered to come to Tollgate House to help with training: Angela Pinder started in late

January that year, working with Helen McCain. She was an ex-employee of GDBA who had shown interest in coming back to work training dogs, and she could live on site with other GDBA staff at Tollgate House.

Further developments during that year were the proposal that we should join Assistance Dogs International, based in the USA, which would lead to better global recognition. David Bennet asked for the charity's name to be changed to 'Dogs for People with Disabilities', but the Trustees rejected the idea, referring to Frances Hay's naming of her new charity. It would be over 20 years before the name change would be acted on. There was a need for disabled people to become their own 'experts' in physical impairment. Disability was defined in 1998 as the disadvantage or restriction of activity caused by a contemporary social organisation that takes little or no account of people who have physical impairments and thus excludes then from participation in the main stream of social activities. Dogs would overcome many of the social restrictions.

The Director of GDBA Operations, Paul Master from Head Office, was appointed as a Trustee to replace GDBA's Brian Moody, who had previously been in charge of the Leamington GDBA training centre. Tollgate House's bungalow, already evacuated by GDBA Staff Training Dept was refurbished and made available, and was to be called Frances Hay House; the commissioned portrait of Frances was to be displayed in the entrance hall there. There were now six dogs training at Leamington and another five were at Exeter under George Cram's care. George had come on the scene after volunteering to make an after-care visit to Bodmin in Cornwall to see Shep, who we will hear more about in the next chapter.

The need for more income with the rapid expansion of dog training was approached in several ways. Five fundraising branches were established, usually at a location where a successful partnership was at work. Oswestry had one such branch and sent in a £1000 cheque after a successful meeting; one of their events was a 'Strawberry Tea' in the house of Millicent Kaye, a branch Patron. Emma, who had suffered a neck fracture in a hang-gliding accident in 1992, was living near the Orthopaedic Hospital in Oswestry, where she had been under treatment. In 1993 she was to come forward to train for an assistance dog at Middlesbrough. In March 1992 she had first come in her wheelchair to a meeting organised by the Oswestry Professional Ladies Club at the Wynnstay Hotel, at which I gave a talk. Other golf clubs' social events were to be another source of donations for Dogs for the Disabled. Young Farmers' Clubs also empathised with the charity; I spoke to a club near Banbury that presented a cheque for Dogs for the Disabled and Helen McCain spoke to the Warwick & Leamington Young Farmers' Club about her work, following an invitation they had sent to the already deceased Frances Hay in October 1991! Banbury Dog Training club held a sponsored swim in 1994 to raise money for us, and later of course a more permanent connection with the town developed.

A variety of money-making events were tried. Debby and David Bennet both took part in the Pet Plan 'Fun Run' at the BSAVA Congress in Birmingham, where a live display of 'helping dogs' on a stand in the commercial exhibition hall was also attended and Helen McCain to promote Dogs for the Disabled. A month or so later, unfortunately, a double booking made by David meant she was sent away to a distant agricultural show on the same Saturday as the GDBA had their annual 'open to the public' puppy show at Tollgate. Circles within the GDBA commented on the poor showing made there by Dogs for the Disabled, with a scout tent and without a presence to show off to the public the lesser dog charity they were financially supporting.

A few weeks later, on the day of the Royal Show, I had to come back to the Leamington GDBA Office to tell David Bennet that his probationary six months would not be extended, so once again we were without a leader.

There were now 33 trained dogs qualified and 25 of them were actively working, while a further nine more were in training, of which five were at Exeter. The Kennel Club Charitable Trust had donated £1500 in recognition of the good image created by showing some of these dogs at work. It was time to bring all the assistance dog organisations in Britain together to discuss future developments and further the need for recognition and access rights. Planning started in July, and an invitation to all known assistance dog groups to come to Tollgate House in September 1992 was responded to by all, with the one exception. Brian Moody was Chairman, as the recently retired Director of Training GDBA. Those attending were George Cochrane of Scottish Canine Consultative Council, Janelle Johnson from Support Dogs Sheffield and Tony Blunt the Director General of Hearing Dogs for the Deaf, who was a Vice Chairman at Assistance Dogs International. Tony had recently attended the 'Animals & Us' conference in Montreal. Val Strong came straight from her holiday venue, joining with Dolores Palmer and Linda Hams, all three of whom did volunteer training under the guidance of John Rogerson, using people's own dogs as assistance dogs. They had been founded in January 1992, and the three trainers all worked well together, each preparing dogs in their own areas, Sheffield, Staffordshire and Northamptonshire.

Each organisation was asked to give a brief talk about the work they were doing. Unfortunately, Tony Blunt was not able to attend to give his report on the international situation which had been planned for the afternoon session, since he was indisposed. I was able to fill in, after the kennel tour of dogs had taken place, with an account of my early army dog training experiences in Melton Mowbray, Egypt and Tripoli. In the lunch hour I was able to speak to Linda Hams on her own; unknown to the others she had been shortlisted for a new post as training manager for Dogs for the Disabled. At earlier interviews she was clearly the best of the three applicants shortlisted, who came from different backgrounds. Linda, as well as being a practical dog trainer, had business experience working for electrical wholesalers, and she had accepted the job a week or so before the assistance dog group meeting. I asked her if the other two knew she was leaving them to work for Dogs for the Disabled and she told me that she had only told them in the lunch break.

In my talk later in the afternoon, I felt uncomfortable knowing that a breakup of the trio of trainers had now occurred. It was the first event held in the charity's new home in the recently-occupied bungalow and it was announced to the dog press that Frances Hay House was fully operational.

Linda Hams started as the General Manager in November that year and brought in new ideas, including different dog breeds to train. An additional part-time secretary, who had previously worked for the GDBA, was engaged to help Debby in the fundraising department. Following the September meeting, the proposal was to form an affiliated organisation to be called the National Association of Support Dogs Organisations (NASDO). There were difficulties even in this name: in the USA they were known as 'Service Dogs'. 'Assistance Dogs' was considered too weak a description. Support Dogs was thought better, but it was already being used by the Sheffield group. A later suggestion was the British Association of Assistance Dogs (BRAD), but it was soon pointed out that this acronym was already being used by an advertising media group.

I mentioned the proposed title to vet Bradley Viner when he took me for interview at the Birmingham veterinary conference. His report was broadcast on London Radio, where a listener pointed out the confusion if the acronym was accepted by the Trustees. The final attempt, accepted by all, was Assistance Dogs United Kingdom

(ADUK), so at last the title of an assistant dog was to be registered for use by organisations training specific tasks to help persons with all sorts of disability.

Progress in assistance dog training could be made in Dogs for the Disabled using their close relationship with the better-financed GDBA charity. The recently-appointed GDBA Executive Director, Julian Oxley, was more sympathetic than his military predecessor and he could see the opportunities if the charities could work side by side. The regular ADUK meetings were often held at Wokingham GDBA head office and gave an opportunity for each charity to appreciate what others were doing.

By the mid-1990s, progress in providing clients with the type of dog they needed was possible with individual training of a chosen dog. The dogs were owned by Dogs for the Disabled but on qualifying were leased out to the disabled person. This arrangement allowed for a dog to be withdrawn and perhaps retrained, returning to the same or another person. The earlier forced withdrawal of Tally from Len would not be repeated. The GDBA still used an older arrangement where the visually-disabled person owned the dog but the white harness (owned by GDBA) could be removed from the owner, preventing the dog being used. It was very rare for these penalties to have to be imposed, but it was necessary to have some form of control in case of misuse or even abuse of a dog.

Linda Hams, as General Manager, compiled a 61-page document early in 1993, described as 'Overview and Three Year Plan', and it included the arguments for and against using 'rescue dogs'. Of the 15 dogs in training none could be called 'abandoned', a word previously used when fundraising. George Cram and Carolyn Bull jointly trained six dogs at Exeter; Lucy Hargreaves had three to train, as well two from Wokingham. Angela Pinder had three dogs at Leamington and Helen McCain had four dogs there too, two ready for matching while two were in early training. Carolyn Fraser had been paid £600 a dog. She trained from her Coventry home, but her work was already phased out. There were five Golden Retrievers, six Labradors, two Labrador crosses, one German Shepherd and another one crossed with a Golden Retriever.

Both Helen and Angela were due to go away in November 1993 for a GDBA-funded visit to the Canine Companions for Independence course in California. In August 1993, Julian Oxley was able to present a paper to the GDBA Council stating that Frances Hay had first approached his predecessor for money in 1987, and now there was a 'sound legal basis' for supporting an established similar charity at an annual cost of £150,000. Their constitution, perhaps dating from the 1930s, allowed for them to help allied charities, which until then had been largely used to respond to blind welfare requests.

The offer was made to allow dogs to be trained in the north of England by using spare kennels at the GDBA Middlesbrough centre. Three trainers were seconded. The Breeding Centre's manager would be available for one day a week and the salary of a General Manager for the first year of the appointment was guaranteed. Julian Oxley said GDBA should intensify their support of the sister charity. Dogs unsuited for guide dog work could be transferred, but using rescue animals in kennels with GDBA dogs would present a problem at the Breeding Centre kennels. By this time dogs obtained from rescue kennels had ceased to be selected for assistance dog training. This Proposal would all cost less than 0.5% of the GDBA's annual expenditure, but it still required the approval of the Charity Commission to direct funds raised for guide dogs to support other assistance dog work.

The search for a new leader was over when Peter Gorbing was engaged in June 1995, through the good offices of the GDBA's selection process. Peter had applied to the GDBA in February 1995 and by good luck his application was brought to the notice of the Trustees of Dogs for the Disabled. He was initially appointed as a Publicity & Fundraising Manager, concentrating on finding more income through fundraising. He worked with Linda Hams, who continued to look after all training matters, helped by Helen McCain, who remained on the staff seconded from the GDBA. Linda had drawn up a three-year plan to increase the number of dogs trained, after having the confidence of backing from the GDBA's additional funding.

There were 39 partnerships working well, mainly located in the centre and the south-west of England. The dogs trained were made up of 31 skilled assistance dogs, with eight dogs classed as companion/social support dogs. The source of the dogs was interesting: at that time 11 dogs had come from rescue kennels, 22 had come from the GDBA as surplus to their needs and four had been specifically 'puppy walked' to train later for Dogs for the Disabled's own use. The list of people who had trained these dogs is also of historical interest: four by Frances Hay, eight by Carolyn Fraser, 10 by Helen McCain, five by Angela Pinder and 10 from the Exeter GDBA centre, trained by George Cram and Carolyn Bull. The use of Middlesbrough for training more assistance dogs would require two additional trainers if the plan could be fulfilled, but this later development eventually proved to be impracticable.

On the fundraising side, a drive to increase regular income was needed. Debby had married and (as Debby Robbins) was to be made Public Relations Officer, allowing Peter Gorbing a free hand to develop new sources. I recruited one of Derek Freeman's former secretaries to catch up on Debby's office work with more branches. This brought a reprimand from Paul Master in the form of a GDBA letter, stating it was done in a 'very amateurish way'. Debby had sported her new assistant to Linda Hams, who must have informed Paul at GDBA Head Office. It seemed petty at the time and perhaps the only time the more bureaucratic charity tried to impose control over the younger and more flexible charity I chaired.

The care of the local branches and the sale of branded goods and souvenirs was given to the newly-appointed Pam Faulkner. This was necessary following previous difficulties with the many different items being ordered at the request of volunteer branches and going 'missing': a stock restriction of only five Dogs for the Disabled's own items would be handled, to allow for tighter stock control. T-shirts and sweatshirts were to be ordered in addition but not to be 'lost'.

The board of Trustees of Dogs for the Disabled had been rearranged so that GDBA-connected persons would continue to have a 5 to 4 voting majority. It was also agreed that I would hand over the chairman's position to Julian Oxley. The arrangement lasted for about 18 months until events brought about a situation where I was again asked to resume the Chairman's role.

By 1994, following the new arrangements, the first training classes to be held in the north of England were commenced. Without any publicity, there was a shortage of suitable northern applicants, so Derek from Coventry and Emma from Shropshire travelled to the Middlesbrough GDBA centre, where there were two rooms adapted for wheelchair users. The two were to associate daily with visually-impaired persons training for their guide dogs, and this arrangement worked well. Three trainers had to travel to Middlesbrough to run the course, Helen McCain, Karen Briggs and Charlotte Mann. It would be many years before applicants from the northern area would require two trainers to be permanently based in Yorkshire; once more potential clients started applying for an assistance do. Linda Ham's position as Training Manager for Dogs for the Disabled was to change. In retrospect this must have been a need for the larger organisation to consolidate its relationship with the younger expanding charity, but events were to unfold which would precipitate a change of direction.

At about this time the Canine Partners organisation was still only just starting to get its trained dogs out. With Nina Bondarenko in charge of Canine Partners for Independence, formerly known as Assistance Dogs for Disabled People (ADAPT), an exchange of information became possible. Nina visited Linda at Tollgate, then Linda was invited to attend CPI's first initial assessment of the four dogs they had trained at Kingsley House in Hampshire. Claire Guest from Hearing Dogs was to attend as the dog assessor, and the day went off well, with the trainers from the three allied charities cooperating and learning about each other.

In September 1994, an unfortunate event occurred after a veterinary surgeon in general practice operated on a dog, Arran. The dog had been working with a client, Tony, who had the disability Duchenne's Muscular Dystrophy. Arran had come from Exeter GDBA with a mild hip disorder but had been trained to help Tony at home. It was understood that after jumping up to the wheelchair, the dog slipped and dislocated a hip. Despite a request for 'conservative treatment' and referral to the orthopaedic department of Bristol Veterinary College, the vet insisted on operating on Arran in his own practice. The dog was euthanased three days later by the veterinary surgeon without anyone first contacting the charity. There was no post-mortem done and the body was immediately removed for cremation the same afternoon following death.

Tony was distressed; he contacted his trainer, George Cram at Exeter, who phoned me immediately he heard of the dog's death. I had no response to my enquiry about what had happened after the operation. There was little that could be done by the charity except quickly train a replacement for Arran at Exeter. Tony's condition meant he had a short life expectancy and Arran should have remained with him much longer.

There was an unresolved situation over the cost of the surgery and possible damages. There had been confusion over the dog's legal ownership, as was shown later. Following a protracted correspondence, in 1999 at Cardiff County Court, the case Kirk v Guide Dogs for the Disabled was heard by District Judge North. After two days of evidence, the case was won for the charity, but when the written judgment was received no costs were awarded by the Judge. The Cardiff barrister's fees were £1431.26, there was my time as attending as witness for Dogs for the Disabled and two road journeys from Leamington to Cardiff, and there was not even compensation awarded for the loss of a trained dog. An appeal by the plaintiff against the findings of the County Court was rejected and the 'Flying Vet', as he wished to be known, has had an interesting subsequent career. I kept a large folder of the correspondence and judgment filed away. A Bristol newspaper report in January 2004 was headed 'Ex-city animal doctor storms out of hearing, bent lawyers to blame, says vet'. By then he had been struck off, in May 2002, following a disciplinary hearing at the Royal College of Veterinary Surgeons after an assault case in 1997 and subsequent court appearances on other charges.

Following the court case findings, the Dogs for the Disabled Trustees agreed it was necessary to define our clients as 'keepers' rather than 'owners' of their assistance dogs which was a point of dispute in the Cardiff legal arguments. A dog would remain owned by the charity, as was stated in the introductory document, and when qualifying the client became a licensed 'keeper'. The wording was never disputed again over who gives consent for a veterinary procedure, as there were always good relations with a sympathetic veterinary profession.

The Trustees said that we should also review our policy of issuing dogs that had previously been diagnosed with hip dysplasia even in its mildest forms. Arran had been obtained from the GDBA with a degree of hip deformity which was considered unlikely to be a disadvantage for a sedentary client who would not take a dog outdoors for activities like jumping obstacles. The decision to defend the original claim for the vet's operation fee for Arran was taken at the Tollgate House offices after legal advice by a Trustee, which I and Linda Hams agreed was necessary to protect Dogs for the Disabled's name.

Chapter 6

A growing independence

Once again the charity was facing problems over where it could work and operate from. The use of Tollgate House as the base was curtailed when the temporary planning permission given for the use of the bungalow as offices was not renewed by the planning authorities. The GDBA also had a need for more kennelling to take in an increasing number of their puppies for boarding and redistribution, as their puppy-walking scheme had expanded. There was the risk of disease being brought into the breeding centre with many puppies at risk. The parvovirus epidemic in the late 1970s hardly touched the GDBA stock, since dispersal of puppies stopped cross-infection, but overcrowding would increase any disease risk.

Julian Oxley, as Chairman, said they would again help us by giving us the use of part of some kennels they were buying at the Old Vicarage, Ryton on Dunsmore, near Coventry. The main purpose of this purchase was to set up a GDBA puppy handling centre, and they would have their own staff living in the roomy vicarage building there. At first there was no office accommodation ready, so it was unfortunate that when Peter Gorbing started work for Dogs for the Disabled, the Trustees had to rent a former railway office where he and Debby would temporarily be based. The rooms at the Deppers Bridge office were on the platform of the main Paddington to Birmingham route, and passing high speed trains coming away from the Harbury Cutting rocked the furniture at intervals. Peter recalls that when he started work there was only a dog bed, a desk with a phone and a chair, but he set about the job until office space was eventually provided at the new Ryton centre.

Towards the end of 1995, we were required to explain our relationship with the GDBA to the Charity Commission. Ian Burr, as a solicitor and a founder Trustee, was authorised to make the reply, explaining Dogs for the Disabled's role in providing assistance dogs in as effective a way as possible. More enquiries were to follow later from the Commission about the relationship.

Once the move of the offices from Tollgate to the GDBA Ryton site was completed in 1997, the work required more office staff. In December 1994, Christine Temple had been appointed Office Supervisor after the resignation of the first secretary, Doreen Cross. Christine had been one of the key people when the organisation was set up. Doreen had loyally stayed on after being relocated from Frances Hay's home office and had maintained a valuable link over the following four years as the charity stabilised its administration.

1994 had also saw the first dogs trained in the north of England, using the GDBA centre at Middlesbrough. By the second half of the 90s, the charity was able to progress. Landmark events celebrated in 1996 were the 100th dog trained and the appointment of the first two apprentices who had to go through the three-year scheme to become qualified assistance dog instructors.

Another appeal for money using BBC's Lifeline was presented by our Vice Patron, Wendy Richard, an enthusiastic supporter. The BBC

TV charity programme appeal showing the assistance dogs at work raised £63,000 in donations, and brought in new supporters. The first application made to the National Lottery Charities Board for a development grant was rejected. We learnt more about the process of application and the challenge was there to make use of the new freedom of competing with the GDBA for funding. Peter Gorbing, whilst still based at the railway platform office, had been appointed as General Manager, and he was asked to prepare for another lottery funding application. There was just one secretary to help him at a time when the salary bill was rising, with a gross income of only £81,813 in the year to cover all training and other costs.

In September 1996, the Charity Commission indicated that they were concerned that the majority of Dogs for the Disabled Trustees were connected to GDBA. The larger charity was required to cease to be a corporate Trustee, and additional Trustees should be appointed who were not GDBA nominees. A retired general practitioner from the Leamington area, and Jane MacDonald, as a client with senior nursing management background, were invited to join the board. Both made valuable contributions and Jane continued as an active Trustee until her death following progressive multiple sclerosis many years later.

The charities involved in preparing assistance dogs, all working together as Assistance Dogs UK, planned a launch to the public at the flagship Marks & Spencer store in Oxford Street, London. Each charity would provide a client and a dog; a Member of Parliament would be there to open the event, early in one morning in February 1996. Full press coverage was arranged and TV cameras could show dogs passing through the food aisles, ignoring the tempting foods at dogs' eye level. The event went ahead early the next year but in the interval, an unexpected exposure of the GDBA's financial state in the national press resulted in long-term changes in the development and growth of Dogs for the Disabled. A number of guide dog owners had been concerned about their own charity's activities and they engaged an accountant to examine the published GDBA annual accounts (all charities have to supply these to the Charity Commission by law). The information available to the public and recorded in the Trustee minutes was that GDBA had assets of £154 million and the guide dog owner group went to a Sunday Newspaper with information that £118 to £120 million was held in investments, whilst property was valued at £54 million. The GDBA justified their reserves, as a blind person might need five or six guide dogs in their lifetime and they had to be able to fund this lifetime commitment they made to the visually disabled. The support that had been given to Dogs for the Disabled was either ignored or never mentioned in the ensuing press investigations, only that ancillary services to the blind were being funded.

The accountants instructed by the guide dog owners' group also found a minor sum of just over £1000 in the GDBA staff mortgage scheme that was demonstrated to be in the Director General's name. It had been overlooked after he had moved house to be closer to the Windsor or Wokingham GDBA office, I was told.

Unfortunately this led to Julian Oxley's unexpected early retirement. In a personal letter to me in November 1996, he wrote he had been 'put out to grass' two years before his intended retirement and expressed his regret that he could not continue the development work following 'short sighted and unjust measures'. He wrote that he had enjoyed his time with Dogs for the Disabled away from the more bureaucratic GDBA and referred to 'the politics of the blind'. He added, 'I also have the greatest respect for what you personally contributed to the development'.

Julian's continued help would have been invaluable, but others felt the situation would be too delicate at a time when we were so interrelated with the GDBA finances. Dogs for the Disabled entered into a new contract, paying £5000 for each dog trained by GDBA staff, the fee to be increased to £7500 for 1997. When Julian was asked to take early retirement in November, it also removed him as Chairman of Dogs for the Disabled and I was asked to take over the post again by the four remaining Trustees. On December 15th 1996, eight years after the first election to find a successor to Frances Hay, I again became Chairman of the Trustees. If it had not been for the investigation of the GBBA finances, Julian could have become the Chairman of Dogs for the Disabled board after his planned retirement. He had been a very good friend to assistance dogs, and one day he could see how all the charities might come together as a single organisation to provide an improved national coverage.

The GDBA had set a target of supporting 5000 guide dog owners by the year 2000. The target was not attainable. The greater use of aids to mobility such as long cane work developed, and dogs were less required to work in congested and stressful situations to help the visually impaired. An increasing proportion of elderly blind were not fit enough to work with a large Labrador Retriever cross. A reorganisation of GDBA under the supervision of the Charity Commission, called the 'Change Project' became necessary. Dogs for the Disabled received approval for their involvement. A Charity Commission statement, now often overlooked, said 'GDBA's support for Dogs for the Disabled has helped to establish it as a successful organisation. GDBA's future role is the provider of direct rehabilitation and mobility services to the blind and partially sighted people. The time is right for Dogs for the Disabled to take its independence'.

1997 was the year of the Lottery Bid for new kennels. The year had started well on January 15th with the press and dog organisations invited to a reception in the Palace of Westminster sponsored by Sir Dudley Smith MP, himself a local dog owner and client of our veterinary practice in Leamington Spa. The assistance dog event was set up around the launch of a dog book written by myself and Neil Ewart, The A to Z of Dog Diseases and Health Problems, published by Ringpress. Invitations were sent out widely to the dog community and the reception adjacent to the House of Commons was attended by guests from the Kennel Club and from the other assistance dog organisations and by a number of veterinary surgeons. It also demonstrated the close cooperation between persons in GDBA and Dogs for the Disabled, since both authors were involved in these allied charities.

Dogs for the Disabled had been training dogs at three centres, Ryton, Middlesbrough and Exeter, and there was a 35% increase in funds raised. Debby Robbins retired when she moved away, having been the first full-time employee. The Blue Cross had recognised Debby's dog Elton as Career Dog of the Year with an award in 1996, thanks to her publicity work for assistance dogs. Peter Gorbing continued as General Manager of the Dogs for the Disabled centre, but he had been away doing some work for the Red Cross charity for several months from February 1998 before returning to work at the Ryton centre. Linda Hams, who by then had joined the GDBA staff, and Peter Gorbing met with the Trustees every month at the Ryton offices to discuss finances and policies. Paul Master, whilst a GDBA Trustee, had encouraged Linda to try training new dog breeds, including two Portuguese Water Spaniels, a Finnish Lapphund and a Springer Spaniel. Purchased from breeders, they were placed in the homes of Dogs for the Disabled puppy socialisers; a Nova Scotia duck-tolling retriever known as 'Toller' for short was also tried.

The office staff at Ryton was increased with Jill and June joining, who ran the office during Peter's absence. I met with them on a weekly basis in between the Trustee regular meetings. An addition was made to help the two new apprentices: a staff training officer, Pauline Hutchinson, who had been transferred by the GDBA to Ryton, set up a training group for more assistance dog trainers. Twenty dogs a year were being trained and it was planned to double the number within a few years. Linda Hams had been offered the post, to be directly employed by the GDBA since they saw her potential in developing dog training; unfortunately this led to her eventual redundancy when the change process required that the GDBA would reduce the number of their training sites and their staff preparing for guide dogs.

After Julian Oxley retired from the Dogs for the Disabled Trustee Board, his experience in chairing the meetings was missed. He said he felt it would be ungracious if he stayed as an independent Trustee at a time when negotiations were still taking place for a phased-out funding coming from the GDBA. The Charity Commission supervised a change programme, but it was was such that GDBA would not want to be seen to be suddenly abandoning their help to the smaller charity.

At one stage it looked as if half the Dogs for the Disabled staff would have to be made redundant, as the salary bill far exceeded the independent fundraising income. A short-term arrangement to continue to occupy the Ryton site, with a rent of £5000 a year, was negotiated. There was an offer made to buy the site at valuation, but six remaining Trustees felt there were too many restrictions if we continued there and a move to a fresh site to train dogs was now necessary. A new application to the National Lottery Board was prepared, and as the reinstated Chairman, I worked on the project with Peter to look for a new site. We were restricted by planning permission requirements as a centre would have to be based on existing boarding kennels that already had permission to keep dogs.

A number of commercial kennels were visited in Warwickshire, in the Coventry area, but all seemed unsuited for our expansion plan. After visiting those advertised in Warwickshire, particulars came in the post for a £365,000 freehold kennel site near Banbury. The kennels were away from our natural development area, as they were on the Oxfordshire–Northamptonshire borders, but they would have good road and rail links to London and the south, to suit visiting clients. Peter went down to look at it, reported favourably and when I was able to go to view it with a disabled friend I agreed that the spacious site had great potential.

I made my first visit to Kathanna Kennels, Banbury, with Jane McDonald, whilst we were still awaiting the National Lottery bid result. We both met the owner, Mrs Robson, who took us into her large five-bedroom bungalow. There was permitted kennelling for 57 dogs and over 30 cats. Nearby was a stable, and a horse ménage and a large hall could both be used in dog training. The price was almost twice the cost of buying the existing Ryton Kennels from the GDBA; there were no reserve funds sufficient for such a property purchase.

We decided to go to the National Lottery with a business plan, something that Peter took up and prepared, with good results. Jane, in her wheelchair, had been able to view the site as a client with her dog Lenny. With her obvious disability she was also able to impress the present owner of the importance of the finding a place to start a national centre for assistance dog work. Jane Macdonald had a forceful personality. She had been assistant registrar for the UK Central Council for Nurses, Midwives and Health Visitors - the profession's regulatory body - when she was diagnosed with multiple sclerosis in 1988. She had appeared on television, showing how in her own home she could use Lenny to help raise herself from the floor, something Mrs Robson remembered when she met Jane.

Whilst we awaited the results of the Lottery application, the delay in being able to make a purchase was causing difficulties for Mrs Robson, the kennels' owner, who wanted to move away further south. She said she had already lost the opportunity to buy one kennel property there through our delays. The asking price of £365,000 was above our valuation, creating uncertainty, as we knew that only 1 in 6 lottery applications was successful. At times we felt we had lost the chance, and she did not get our decision to purchase for almost a year. Fortunately no other purchasers were interested in the site, which was close to the M40 motorway but limited by being in the green belt. The industrial development area for Banbury was on the opposite south side of the motorway. There was a late enquiry to use the site for radio communication masts, but there was no other offer to buy the dog kennels.

The application process for capital to purchase Kathanna Kennels became the next focus of office activities. The purchase of the site was at the valuation of £365,000, with additional money required for building a new office and accommodation block costing £235,000. Access work for the kennel site would cost £22,000, and some refurbishment of the bungalow would also be needed for staff living in. The existing training hall, 48ft x 33ft, could be used at once, but with more dogs and people on the site a new sewage disposal system was necessary, costed at £32,500, with equipment & contingency estimated at £30,000. The Lottery were asked to cover all items except the last, making the total needed £555,000.

An application form requiring the Chairman's signature as a Declaration of Intent was signed by me on September 24th 1997. The income for the year ending Dec 1998 was £344,334, down from £431,960 in the previous year, whilst expenditure was £308,253. There were only four directly employed staff, while dog training and expenses cost £159,332, reduced from £348,846 in the previous year, as the wage bill had been cut. Dogs were all being trained by the GDBA employed staff, at a contract price of £5000 paid as each dog qualified. A building development fund, largely collected from legacies over several years, stood at £200,712 and was designated for the new building. One legacy involved selling a house at Filey, which was in dispute until eventually probate was granted that added to the building fund.

The Banbury architects engaged were a wise choice and they later obtained an award for their building design. The planning applications were made and building contractors were asked to tender, all at the same time. In March 1998, the charity gained possession of the Banbury site after Mrs Robson vacated her bungalow. Trainer Louise Hart and her husband moved into the bungalow and provided the site security; they occupied their quarters with a £50 a week licence being paid. Building work was to start in May and to finish by November 26th 1999. The training of dogs continued under Helen McCain's leadership. The Exeter centre was being phased out by the GDBA for all training. As George Cram, who was based there, was over GDBA's retirement age, he could continue with after-care client visits, but Caroline was regrettably made redundant. At Middlesbrough, the sole trainer, Karen, was brought back to the Ryton base, as at that stage the demand from the north had not developed as expected and money was short.

Peter and Helen drew up guidelines for future dog training which meant increasing the puppy scheme and keeping dogs in people's homes out of kennels, whenever possible. A semi-intensive training period of nine months for each dog would provide dogs ready to qualify at 22 months. These slightly older dogs, after training with the client, would wait until three months after the class was completed to qualify as registered assistance dogs.

Client selection involved looking for younger active people – Wendy Morrell was one such person, an example of how a dog could enhance the life of a person in a wheelchair. The trained dogs were to do more than act as companions for the housebound but would encourage access to the workplace and social activities. An instructor in a 24 month-period could place 15 clients, so that with five full-time Dogs for the Disabled Instructors, the plan would allow 75 clients a year to be trained. Unfortunately such a development plan took a long time to reach fulfilment, and there were many setbacks; the target for the number of dogs trained a year was not reached until eight years later.

The plan of training from a new centre was assessed as feasible by accountants who had also reported on the cost of the system of external training by contract. Outsourcing using the salaried GDBA trainers, if based on providing 20 dogs at £7500 each and three dogs at £2500, would need £157,500 a year with the additional costs of rearing puppies and making after-care visits. Greater public awareness of the benefits of assistance dogs was required to improve the charity's profile. The Labrador Kandy, with young Jamie, had become Companion Dog of the Year at London WAG Show 1998. Their picture was used on the publicity posters and emphasised his search for work following his disabling cycle accident when out delivering early morning newspapers.

Another dog that gained media attention was Yvette, a Golden Retriever which had come from the Cardiff Guide Dog Centre. She was trained by Helen McCain for a Birmingham lady, whose disability of cerebral palsy (CP) led to a good working partnership, and she would go out with Yvette giving talks; the high point in the talk I attended was when Yvette helped her undress! Others with CP were subsequently to benefit from dogs. Ever since the mid-90s it had become a question of finding out where dogs could most be of use to help with disabilities, especially where a potential client had was no previous experience of dog ownership.

The 150th partnership was completed by Sarah Carr and Jade, a replacement for her first dog Zac, and she was also used in publicity events. The Liverpool Victoria Society, as sports sponsors, had picked Steve Davis to play for Dogs for the Disabled charity at the Derby Snooker Tournament. Steve progressed through several rounds, which raised £13,000; he met Sarah, who was there with Linda Hams, but confessed he was not really a great dog lover! Blue Peter kept up their connection with the charity too, and had visited Ann Greenwood after she had her new dog Baron in Cornwall.

Chapter 7

Successes in the new millennium

As the new century and millennium began, Dogs for the Disabled's work was beginning to make an impact in the disability world, since there was general satisfaction with the use of dogs trained to help with disabilities. In November 2000, I received a letter from a client in County Durham about a dog trained in the North of England:

'Dear Mr Lane and Fellow Trustees, it is now a year since I was 'partnered' with my dog, Bridie, and I feel I must write and say a heartfelt thank you. It was only pure luck that I found out about Dogs for the Disabled when I was actually pestering the Middlesbrough centre for a retired guide dog to keep me company during the day when my husband and family were not at home. Never did I think I'd be fortunate enough to acquire a constant companion who offers unconditional love, security around the house and helps with difficult tasks around the house. Besides working for me she has brought nothing but joy to the entire family and is helping them to cope with my disabilities. I also feel I have to say how impressed I've been with the care and attention from everyone in DFD, especially my instructors Karen Jones and Duncan Edwards. Such commitment and dedication in young people is both refreshing and admirable. I had hoped to meet you in September but the fuel crisis prevented it, so I look forward to getting down to Oxford some time in the future. Till then kindest regards, and all the best for 2001!

　- Anita Knowles.'

A letter like this was very encouraging and it was unfortunate that I was never able to meet the lady. It did mean a lot to the instructors and other staff when people appreciated the extra effort they were putting into their training with the dogs.

Another satisfied client amongst the group of persons trained in the first decade of Dogs for the Disabled was Ann, who after 26 years still continues to work with her fifth dog. She is now the living pioneer of the successful application of the use of dogs to help with disabilities. She recently told me that assistance dogs had 'changed my life completely" and 'let me get the horses back'. Ann, when younger, was a teacher in a school in Kent, but with a problematic health condition she had moved to live in Cornwall; after a back condition deteriorated she had to give up full-time work. She had always been used to having horses, both riding and driving with a trap (a two-wheeled cart). I asked her how she came to have her first dog in 1988 and she said it was after seeing a TV Blue Peter programme with Amanda's dog Poppy at work that she had wanted to find out more about the new charity. She had recently lost her own pet Jack Russell terrier and was no longer able to go with her wheelchair to get to the nearby stables where her horse and a donkey were kept. She had phoned up Frances Hay at Kenilworth and after a friendly discussion was told there could be a 'chance'. She was not to know that Carolyn Fraser, living in Coventry, had found a Collie abandoned on the side of the motorway and was then training it up for assistance work. She called the dog 'Shep', and the first task was getting the pads of all four feet healed, as they had been worn down to raw flesh, perhaps from trying to follow a moving car after being dumped on the roadside.

The training of Shep in Carolyn's home had taken about a year, with a slow improvement in the dog's confidence, but Shep showed a willingness to learn new tasks. He was taught to walk close beside the old pram she had kept in order to get used to a wheelchair moving beside him. The next thing Ann heard was that Shep was ready to come to her, having progressed well after living with Carolyn's family. Shep was never put into kennels throughout training.

In the early days there were no vehicles used by the charity, so it was arranged that Carolyn would bring Shep by train from Coventry to Bodmin accompanied by her two children; they would all stay in a bed & breakfast in Nanstalon village for a week. Word got round the villages about this wonder rescue dog and instead of Ann's mother on her own meeting the visitors at Bodmin Station, the local press and BBC Radio Cornwall were out on the platform as well. Carolyn's family had not expected such a reception on a 'holiday trip'.

All went well with the interviews on arrival. Carolyn had worked for Guide Dogs for the Blind as a trainer before her marriage and was able to answer all the questions about how a dog was trained and what Shep would do. Later when TV South West came with television cameras to film Shep following the first radio interview, the home training was progressing well. Such publicity was welcome at that stage for the developing charity and it later led to Shep's appearance on a national children's TV programme.

There were some unexpected problems in the first home training week. One of the tasks Shep had been trained for was to help with shopping and carry a basket in his mouth. When on the second day asked Ann 'Should we go shopping now?' Shep was taken down the village street besides the wheelchair with Ann to enter a small cottage village store. Carolyn was shocked as she looked round the interior and exclaimed 'is this it? When I trained Shep for this, we used Coventry Marks & Spencers'. A little retraining, with the grocer filling the basket from a shopping list, then handing it over to Shep to carry up the road, was not too difficult.

The greater problem was only seen after Carolyn returned home at the end of the week. Since Shep had so firmly attached himself to her, he 'fell apart' and forgot most of what he had learnt. On reporting to Frances in Kenilworth about the situation, there was no possibility of sending someone again 400 miles to look into the problem. Carolyn spoke to Ann on the phone and told her not to worry about Shep but just to 'enjoy him'. Fortunately George Cram, an experienced guide dog trainer based at Exeter who I had known when we were both at the Leamington Spa guide dog centre was able to offer his help. When told of the problem, George was able to come to Bodmin by car from the Exeter centre, as he was doing aftercare visits to guide dog owners in Cornwall. With a little confidence building, Shep returned to performing his trained tasks.

Ann found Shep liked pulling at things and he helped her by pulling off her socks at night. Visiting the horse stables, Shep could pull a rope to open the farmyard gate once Ann released the latch. Closing the gate was the next task Shep learnt, by jumping at a board on the gate to push it until it clicked shut. As time went on, Ann could get Shep to fetch items for horse grooming and then help with the placing of the rugs on the horse's back and bringing the girth under the horse between its legs to be fastened by Ann. All of this was eventually shown on national TV as an example of what an assistance dog could do for people in wheelchairs. Such publicity was valuable in demonstrating what Dogs for the Disabled was all about.

Individual training was available for the many differing needs of persons in wheelchairs. Shep next won a competition for West of

England's 'best loved dog', which led to his next journey from the West Country to attend the national finals at the Hilton Hotel in Park Lane, London. A car firm in Exeter loaned a Land Rover and Ann with her friend Pauline drove the whole distance to London, at a time when there were no fast roads out of Cornwall.

Stopping at Cheltenham for a break, they met their first obstacle. The Service Station café shop said no, they could not bring their dog in, but they were saved by the young waitress, who called out 'but that's the dog off Blue Peter that was carrying things!'. The café manager relented and they got their refreshment.

In London, Shep only got the runner up's prize, but after the event was over, they were taken into a side room to meet The Princess Royal, who not only wanted to know what the dog could do but became even more involved with Ann when she heard about Shep's work with the horses. Ann was able to talk about June the pony and the companion donkey she kept, as well as about her assistance dog. Ann also remembered that they talked about Zara, who 'was only little then'. Later there were TV appearances on ITV's 'Good Morning' at the lock cottage studio in East London where Shep showed how he could retrieve a mobile phone dropped on the floor. Another dog there, which had won first prize as best-loved dog, was almost completely ignored.

Later on Anthea Turner, as a Patron of Dogs for the Disabled, visited Ann and her 'marvellous dog' in Cornwall. The TV cameras filmed the horses with Shep and also showed how Ann would go to the village primary school once a week to teach music. Blue Peter later showed how it was necessary for the schoolchildren to bring out two metal channels to make a ramp for Ann to get up the school steps in her wheelchair. When Shep went to a show at the Wokingham guide dog centre, they had got Ann a pony and trap to drive in and Shep was running loose besides the wheels in the demonstration arena, which impressed the crowd.

After several years of fame, unfortunately Shep developed a sound hypersensitivity or 'shyness'. At the stables, if a gate banged in the wind, he would rush off home and hide. George Cram said it couldn't go on and then started looking for a suitable ex-guide dog as a replacement. With nothing suitable at the GDBA Exeter kennels, one of their trainers there, the husband of Caroline Bull, had gone to attend a GDBA development meeting on the Wirral. He heard about a German Shepherd which had been returned there as a guide dog but had not been on offer to the Exeter centre. The dog, Baron, was unsuited to that type of guide work and his puppy walkers would take him back as a pet. Baron would have to be collected for Dogs for the Disabled's use. Fortunately a GDBA staff member was going up to the north west to see her parents, so she was able to pick up Baron and bring him straight to Ann for further training. Caroline Bull had come to work full time for Dogs for the Disabled as a GDBA Exeter seconded trainer and was able to give support to Ann with training her new dog at home in Bodmin. Baron also appeared on Blue Peter, and Ann remembers he was filmed on a freezing cold day visiting the local post office. Baron would go out with Ann driving her pony and trap and he would obediently run beside the wheel and was then allowed out without a lead on Bodmin Moor.

Baron met the Queen when she visited the Exeter guide dog centre for their centenary. Ann remembers that when all the dogs were placed in a line, Baron sat up obediently with his ears raised up over his head. Her Majesty's comment to Ann was 'that is some big dog' and he behaved impeccably. Baron worked well and was retired at 10 years of age.

Ann's next dog, Joel, a German Shepherd, proved less suitable, and after quite a short time he had to be retired early as there was an incident with a group of children; he actually bit a child by accident and was withdrawn from work. The school and the parents understood, as the children were very excited at seeing the animals for the first time. There was then a wait that left Ann isolated and the replacement Kyrie came from the Exeter centre, where George and Caroline were then preparing a number of assistance dogs. Kyrie was donated by the Poole supporters' group and the puppy socialiser there did some horse work too, as they knew he was probably going to Ann. Kyrie was qualified as the last dog to be trained at Cleve House Exeter by Caroline Bull before she was made redundant on the GDBA staff as part of the 1995 downsizing reorganisation.

The next replacement dog for Ann had to come down from Banbury, where he had been in training. Yoshi, her present dog, was trained by Sara. 'Lovely girl, damned good dog trainer, a cracking dog trainer,' Ann said after she received Yoshi some four years ago. Sara and Duncan had brought two dogs down to Cornwall. The other was a black Labrador which took one look at the horses and 'took off', but Yoshi was an instant success. 'He was too hyper for others, but I work him from 7.30 until 10 at night' she said. Ann goes up to see her horses at the nearby stables three times a day. If she does a walk, it's six or eight miles. 'He has to do his running for me,' she says. 'They've lost the aftercare officer and it's not as easy as it was when they came out from Exeter for aftercare visits. Yoshie goes to the library van to collect the books and runs down the steps with the bag in his mouth. Anything involving bending down he does for me'.

The Friesian mare at the stables came over from Holland and the five-year-old horse was a gift from Ann's mother, who died early in 2014. She in her time had been a great supporter of Dogs for the Disabled, going out giving talks and collecting donations for the charity.

When Ann received her first trained dog, she approached her local vicar and requested a special service of thanksgiving! The Vicar of St Stephen's gave his prayer and eulogy: 'Dear Lord we thank you for giving the thought to Frances Hay that dogs could be trained to help those who are disabled. We thank you that she followed this up and began the work of Dogs for the Disabled. We ask Lord that you will continue to help them in this work, giving strength and patience to those who train these dogs, and joy and support to those who will be helped by them. Through Jesus Christ our Lord'.

Within months of that church service, Frances Hay died, but perhaps she had these words in her mind before she passed away on December 22nd 1990.

The publicity about Shep also led to many requests for dogs from people in the south west of England. The opening of the second Dogs for the Disabled centre resulted from that demand; after it opened in Exeter, in the kennels provided by the GDBA, we were able to cover the west of England and South Wales. The unit worked well, with only occasional visits of the two trainers from Warwickshire.

In September 1994 an Exeter-trained dog, Buster, was matched with a Bristol multiple sclerosis client, and this indicated a possible location for a future Dogs for the Disabled base. Following the eventual closure of Cleve House in Exeter by the GDBA, there was no local support for the south west until a centre was opened at Weston Super Mare, later to be moved to Bristol.

Possibly the charity's lack of a permanent home, until Banbury was fixed as the central training facility, meant that clients were not always supported as well as they might have wanted. George Cram had taken Helen McCain to meet Ann at Bodmin in March 1991. Later Helen was officially seconded from GDBA to move from Exeter to live at Tollgate House, where six kennels on the edge of the main block were reserved for Dogs for the Disabled's use. Exeter stayed as a productive training centre with George for most of the early years. With greater involvement with the GDBA and the success of a combined training centre working side by side at Exeter, there was next an opportunity to train dogs in the North of England, where the requirement for more guide dogs was falling. The first class held by Dogs for the Disabled at Middlesbrough GDBA centre was on July 1st 1994. I had spent some time with Derek Coyle, a former builder, who was restricted to a wheelchair after a roofing accident 10 years previously. Aged 32, he was attending the Sports Centre for the Disabled in Coventry when he heard about our charity. It was a time when with the help of the guide dog organisation the charity was expanding into new areas to cope with the demand for dogs. At the GDBA Centre in Middlesbrough, several ground floor student bedrooms had been converted to make them wheelchair accessible and a small fenced courtyard provided outside the French windows, where a dog could be released. Although Derek had three young children at home, he willingly volunteered to go to the north east centre to be trained with a dog if it meant he could get a dog sooner.

The Middlesbrough centre was built on a site on a housing estate previously used as a Roman Catholic Secondary School. One of the guide dog owners trained there complained about the 'wide mouth roads', meaning that the pre-war style housing estate did not have junctions with crossings at right angles to each other. Derek said he found the course 'hard going' at first, being away from home.

Emma was the other student on the class. She had travelled up from Oswestry for her dog Ben; they were the 66th and 67th dogs to qualify as assistance dogs. Outside the centre there were no nearby shops. An often-repeated anecdote was that on one training class, a blind man pushed one of our disabled clients in his wheelchair so they could both reach the local pub further into the estate - a very practical illustration of how guide dog owners and dogs for the disabled recipients could support each other in their various needs!

Before Derek had his new dog, Cherry, he would not go out on his own at all. He said if he went into the city he had swing doors let go onto him in his chair, people would be embarrassed at seeing him and nobody spoke to him, often avoiding eye contact. He told me he thought people had seen TV programmes where people in wheelchairs were always portrayed as bitter and twisted, so they would not speak to him. When he had the dog, it all changed; she gave him a lot of confidence. The visible jacket Cherry wore at work informed people about the partnership and helped to break down the barriers with other people.

In the home, the dog was a great success with his children, who all wanted to be involved in helping to care for it. He would go to pick up the children from school in his wheelchair, and all the other children loved Cherry, calling her 'the disabled dog'. There was even a stranger situation where someone accused him of having a guide dog when there was nothing wrong with his sight!

With the relocation from Tollgate to Ryton on Dunsmore in 1997, Derek in Coventry was able to get close support. The National Lottery award of £597,595 in the summer of 1998 was followed by a search for new premises, and eventually it led to Dogs for the Disabled's move away from outside Coventry to Banbury, much further away from his home.

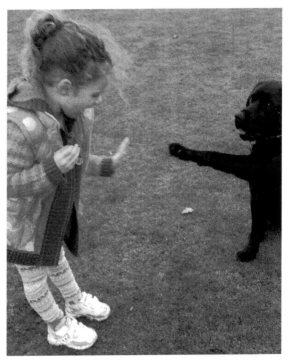

Lucy goes paw to paw

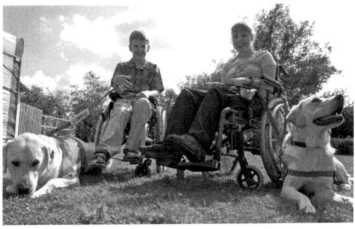

First child teams - Kayleigh, Tom, Vicky and Viggo

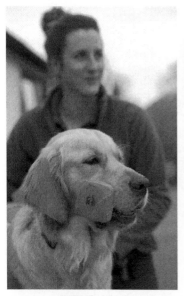

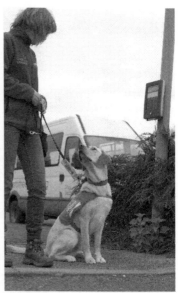

DFD Training   Dogs for the Disabled taskwork

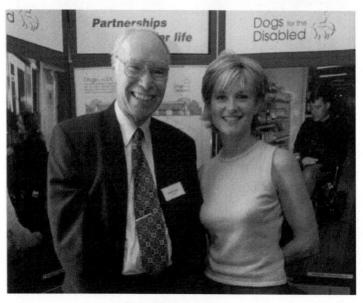

Dick with Anthea Turner

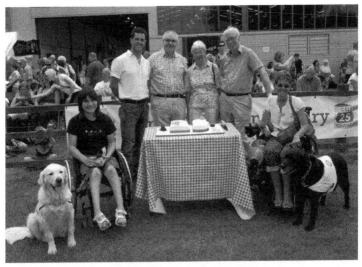

25 years - the three chairpersons

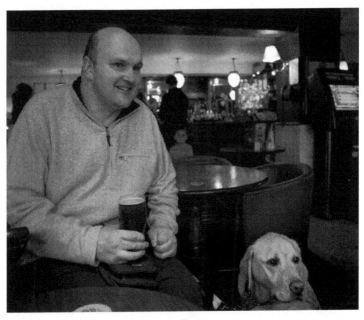

Andy, Trustee

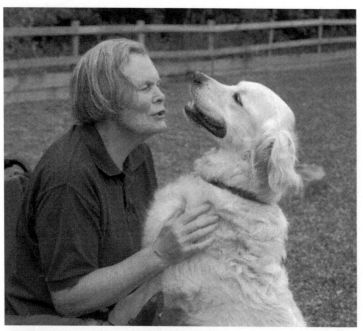

Anne with Yoshi

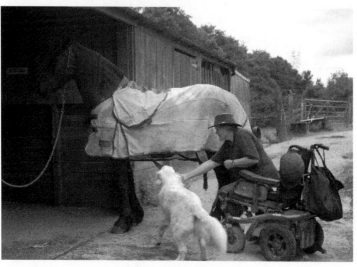

Anne with Yoshi at her stables

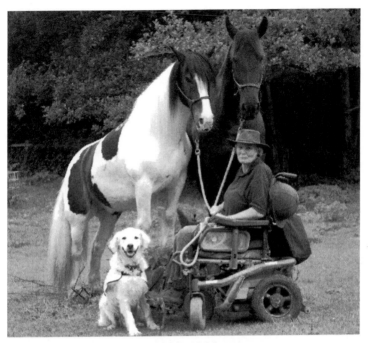

Anne with Yoshi & horse

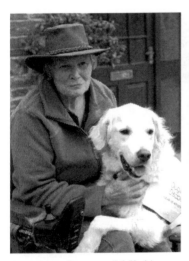

Anne Greenwood & Yoshi

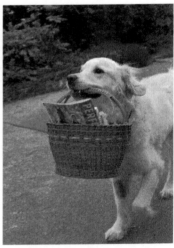

Yoshi carrying the shopping

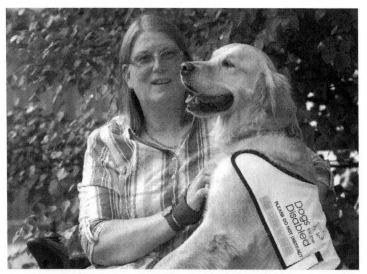

Wendy with Udo

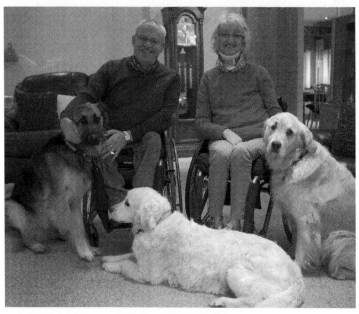

Byron and Sue Harvey

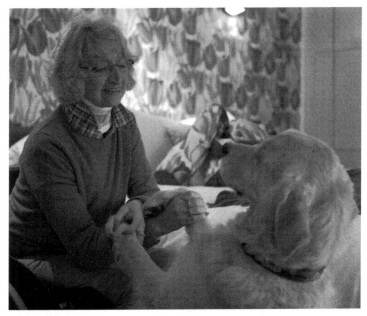

Sue Harvey

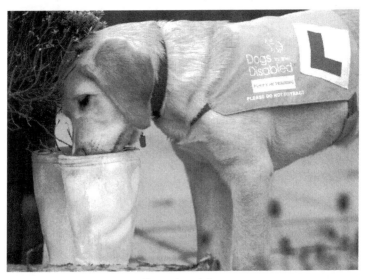

Puppy in training

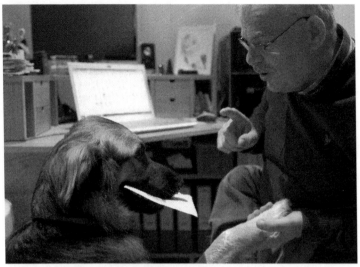

Byron and Ziggy

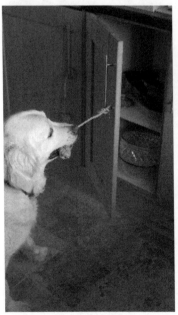

Yoshi doing taskwork

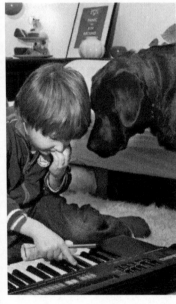

PAWS family - Kristina's son Jude
and Claude

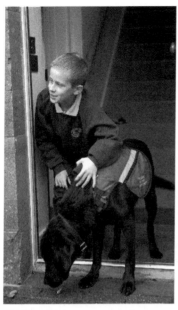

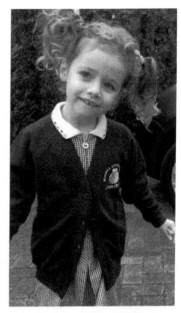

Eddie and Harmony, an autism team   Lucy ready for school

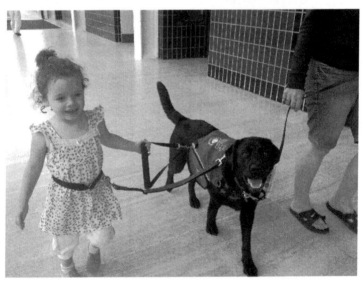

Lucy with Gunner

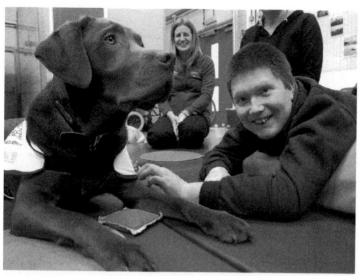

School Dog - Stocklake Park School

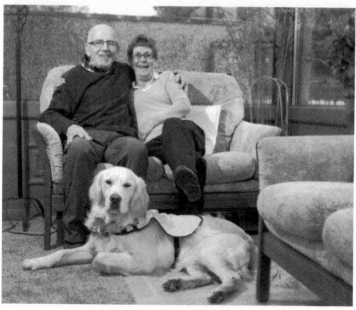

Frank and Maureen with dementia dog Oscar

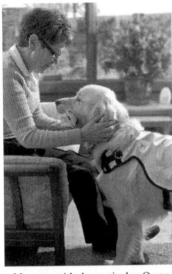

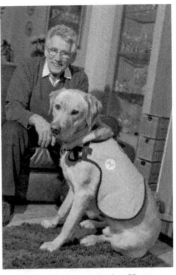

Maureen with dementia dog Oscar   Ken with dementia dog Kaspa

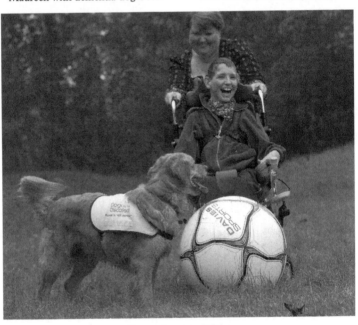

Lorna, Jason and Zeke

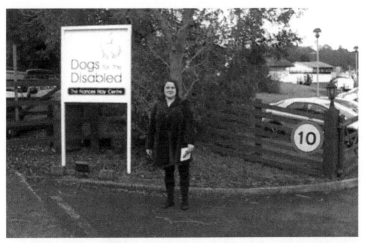

Banbury HQ, Dogs for the Disabled

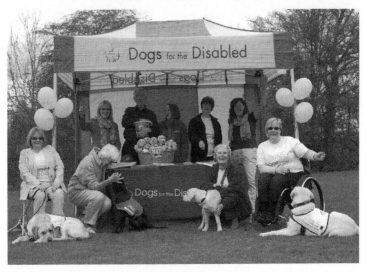

Comunity fundraisers

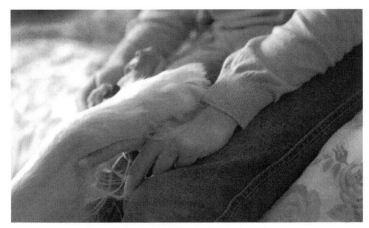

Paw at work

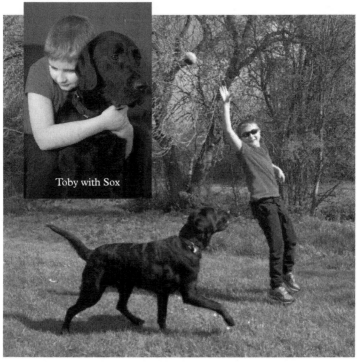

Toby with Sox

Toby at play with Sox

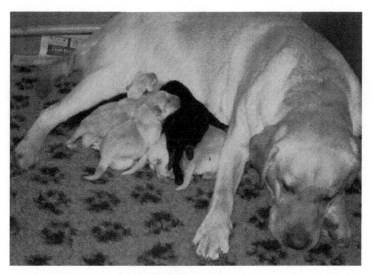

Brood bitch Daisy with pups

Chapter 8

Banbury: more dogs trained by Dogs for the Disabled

With the move to the new site just outside Banbury town, there was a continuing need for a greater local awareness of the charity, to encourage donations and to find volunteers to socialise puppies. Northamptonshire was the county in which the new centre was located, but the area was not associated with any dog-based charity, unlike some of the adjacent counties. Oxfordshire had Hearing Dogs for the Deaf at Aston Rowant, later moving to Chinnor in the Chilterns, and Warwickshire was where GDBA had centres in Leamington Spa and Bishops Tachbrook.

The position of Patron of the Charity was accepted by the Marquess of Hertford. Helen Haighton, a veterinary surgeon friend and supporter of the charity, who lived near Alcester, made the first contacts at the Marquess' home, Ragley Hall. He had wished to visit the Ryton kennels before the move, then after Dogs for the Disabled occupied the Banbury site, he later came to plant a tree in the field next to the newly-built office block. After the planting ceremony, I offered to push his wheelchair over the rough field grass back to the tarmac road, which nearly led to the loss of another Chairman, the uneven surface being harder to push over than my strength would allow, until we finally reached the paved path!

During the continuing work at Banbury site, Martin from the architect's firm worked closely with Peter, visiting the site frequently as the contractors made good progress in the summer. Anthea Turner, as Vice President, came to Banbury town for a press launch promotion and was then driven to see the building site. A battered Portakabin used by the workmen was partly cleared and she was invited to see the kennel plans. I well remember her gallantly picking her way over broken bricks and other debris in the yard in her high-heeled fashion shoes to reach the site office. She took it in good part and had that easy manner of getting builders to talk as soon as she met them. She was interested in what the dogs could do and told me of early experiences of helping a younger member of her own family to get round in a wheelchair. Unfortunately, when Anthea's personal life took a sharp change, for a period she was not making public appearances, so her star quality was not available to the charity.

Another legal situation was encountered, this time to the charity's advantage. The building works at Banbury were nearly completed in 1999: payments had been made at each stage direct to the building contractor without VAT being added. Customs and Excise agreed the site was for a 'Welfare Service' so the building work should be zero rated. It was ruled that if a nominal charge of £1 was taken from the client when the dog qualified in exchange for a licence, then tax would not be charged. A considerable sum was saved and the whole building project remained within budget.

The following year, just before the final stages of the work, the contractor declared himself bankrupt, and another firm had to be called in to complete the final stages. The bankruptcy hearing was some months later. It also led to a reduced payment being required for some of the final stages of the building work.

The move from Ryton kennels to Banbury was completed quickly. Dogs were brought into the kennels and the staff were able to appreciate the facilities, with more office space and the large indoor training area. The site was situated just north of the M40 motorway in a green belt area, so no other industrial expansion threatened the rural feel of the training facility. Before the move took place, knowing what had occurred when Hearing Dogs moved into a Yorkshire village and then had restrictions put on their kennel use through neighbours' objections, I walked round the local householders on a Sunday afternoon knocking on doors to explain the use of the site. Previously as Kathanna boarding kennels it was receiving stray animals from local authorities, and I explained that our dogs would be far quieter and training would be done on site in the hall or in the centre of Banbury for town experience. There was only one planning objection that related to the proposal for a National Training Centre. We had to explain to the South Northamptonshire authority that our title did not mean we would be keeping hundreds of dogs for training.

George Newns wrote to me to say that opening the new training centre was 'a fulfilment of Frances' dreams', but there was still much more work to do once the centre was opened. It was a unanimous decision by the Trustees and others working there that when the building was completed it was to be known as the Frances Hay Centre. It was a great pity the missing portrait in oils could not have been hung in the entrance, but a photo montage from a colour slide I had kept was the next best thing, since the portrait had gone for ever.

Although the training hall next to the kennels was an asset, it was uninsulated. It needed the concrete floor surface improved and the further expenditure of £25000, which also included replacing old window frames. Once completed, the hall could be used as a good facility for assistance dog training. The work on the hall had been largely completed by June 2001 and had been finished under budget. Fortunately, a single donation of £125,000 and a legacy of £30,000 made fitting out the centre possible. A minibus was acquired as a used vehicle from LDV, to enable dogs and clients to be taken into Banbury town during their training. The BBC's Lifeline TV appeal in March 2000 soon added to available funds.

Dogs for the Disabled was entering a new phase, and the management board was strengthened by inviting Peter Helmore and Jerry Brownlee to become Trustees. They both had commercial experience, Peter as a Banbury bank manager and Jerry for his Kennel Club contacts, and they would give valuable advice to the charity in the years ahead. The puppy socialising scheme set up to provide dogs suitable for assistance dog training had 17 puppies at walk and there was even talk that one day we would breed our own puppies rather than relying on known breeders to supply puppies when most needed.

A mission statement was devised stating, 'Dogs for the Disabled provides professionally trained dogs which enable disabled people to be independent by building mutually beneficial partnerships which respect the needs of both client and dog'. As a person who had had her first assistance dog in December 2000 and then trained with her second dog in 2010, Wendy was able to add her experiences of how the charity had progressed in looking after the needs of wheelchair users. Before her accident she had been teaching mathematics and had lectured and been an examiner, she told me. She lived at Bury St Edmunds and one of her hobbies was flying a private aircraft, which might have been considered a hazardous pastime, but her main hobby of archery would have been considered much safer. As a national archery record holder in the 1990s, she had attended the competition venue in Birmingham where the selection of competitors for the European Indoor Championship was to take place. Whilst awaiting her turn in the outdoor arena in the archery area she had suffered a catastrophic injury when hit from behind by a mis-thrown metal discus. The missile struck her across the back of her neck and she recalled nothing of this in the following days until she woke up in the neurological ward of a hospital. Rendered unconscious by the blow, she had at first been taken to a medical room and the hour's delay before the ambulance was called did not speed her treatment. She learnt later that there had been concern by those in the medical room that she would be unable to drive herself home in her car, once she came round. The injuries to the neck bones and spinal cord could not be seen externally.

With regard to her subsequent treatment, it was fortunate that when she had been taken unconscious into the hospital they had found in her back pocket a receipt for an insurance policy for any accident or injury during the event. She had purchased the insurance the same morning as part of the fee for entering the competition. This made a tremendous difference to Wendy in the way her treatment level could be continued into the long subsequent rehabilitation process. Wendy said the NHS physiotherapy and treatment was good, but there was little psychological support for her changed lifestyle. She moved into a bungalow more suited to a wheelchair user, in a pleasant semi-rural area near the south coast.

Throughout this time there was an ongoing court case over who was liable for the injury she had sustained. The hearing of her case, Morrell v Owen, for negligence by the organisers from 1993 was not completed until 1997, with the insurers eventually paying out a substantial sum for her permanent disability. The judgment was that the organizers of a sporting event had a duty of care in sports stadium, as was reported in the Times law report, and it is still referred to in cases involving sports injuries. The organizers of a sporting event for the disabled had a greater responsibility than would be the case for an organizer of a similar event not involving disabled persons, the Judge said.

Some time later, Wendy saw a TV programme involving dogs and disabled people, and realised that a dog could be of help to her in her new situation. It was only after the first year undergoing treatment in her paralysed condition that Wendy first heard of assistance dogs working beside people in wheelchairs in England. She made enquiries in January 1999 from the organizations training such dogs and decided that the course offered by Dogs for the Disabled, who were soon to move from Warwickshire to Banbury, was the one most suited to her needs. Unfortunately, unknown to her, there were cutbacks and possible staff redundancies during the enforced reorganization and on applying for a dog, she was told the application list had been closed. Applying next to Canine Partners, she was quickly called for interview at Petersfield, only to be told she was unsuited for a dog. She says she was told that her voice was not assertive enough (since the neck injury had affected her speech) and that at that time they were only taking clients who were using motor-powered wheelchairs for training with dogs, not the hand-propelled ones she was used to.

Wendy was not easily deterred. When she reapplied to Dogs for the Disabled after nine months in September1999, she was told that since she was now living in Dorset she could have a dog issued from the Exeter Centre, which was a lot closer than Ryton near Coventry. Caesar was trained by Jo Parkinson, who was based at the GDBA Centre, and she could travel daily from Exeter to see that Caesar was suited to Wendy's requirements. Until then Wendy had been reluctant to go out alone. She still had impaired speech from the injury, and people and neighbours were sympathetic but curious to know how she had been in an accident that left her paralysed. She felt there was an air of disapproval or even disbelief that she could have been hurt by just going to attend a sporting event.

When Caesar came, she found in the first weeks that she had to raise her voice to give the right commands and directions when

Caesar was asked to retrieve items. She implied that Caesar had improved her speech far more quickly than the work of a speech therapist. Her increased confidence and clearer speech led to her being invited to speak in London at an event about assistance dogs convened at Westminster to tell parliamentarians about guide dogs and how the newer types of assistance dogs were working. Although Wendy had not been involved in the new training facility in Banbury, with Caesar she could qualify from Exeter on December 7th 2000.

A new world was about to open for her. She had been able to have domiciliary training with Caesar being brought to her home, where the final stages of assistance dog training could take place, so there was no need to travel to the Frances Hay Centre. In her own words: 'Slowly as we began to trust each other, our world got bigger. All the time together, we'd pop our toes outside the comfort zone and together we found freedom. Caesar took his work as an assistance dog very seriously and was always ready to help, but he never lost his love of the outdoors and was just as capable of coming home as black as any dog!

'Caesar was a joyful soul and always had a cuddle to spare – he knew instinctively how to work a room full of people. Over the years he has got me out of some very sticky situations. He once chased away a naked masked man who nearly assaulted me. He would fetch and carry for my dad when he was poorly and staying with us. He was self-taught in alerting me to epileptic seizures and intuitively knew when my friend Karen was unwell. Caesar's alerts were the inspiration for Karen getting her own medical alert dog, since he always knew before something was about to go wrong. No matter how much I write, I will never be able to explain how Caesar became a terrific support as an assistance dog as well as a friend... he was one of those dogs where to know him was to love him'.

I had first met Wendy on a one-to-one basis, at Crufts' Dog Show in Birmingham. Wendy had come along with Caesar as a spectator and whilst she was visiting the Charity's display stand, I was able to fall into an easy conversation with her. We became immediate friends and I told her of a conference in Glasgow I was going to later that year. Caesar, as the model assistance dog, could now travel everywhere with Wendy, so she had no difficulty in getting from her home in the south to the Scottish Conference hotel situated beside the River Clyde. I was attending a Course at Myerscough College in Lancashire at that time, so I was able to drive to Glasgow from Lancashire in the late afternoon after the day course lectures. I was slightly delayed and having arranged to meet Wendy, I found her already in the hotel foyer with Caesar as she got to the IAHAIO Conference site earlier than me. I suggested meeting her over dinner later on as I wanted to check into my room. Fortunately I thought it first best to book a table in the hotel restaurant, as it had a two-tiered floor and the upper section would not have been accessible.

When I informed the waiter I wanted a table for two and a suitable place for access for a wheelchair and a dog, I was firmly told 'We do not allow dogs in this restaurant'. In fact the first table I was offered was up a small flight of steps and fresh from my recent lecture on access rights, I spoke with authority to the waiter that he was not allowed by law to discriminate and he could not exclude a registered assistance dog under the new European laws. As this was the first evening of an international conference on assistance animals, I felt I had struck a blow that would benefit other conference delegates who might want to eat there with their dogs, especially those who would arrive later with assistance animals. Hotel management obviously got the message and there were no further difficulties. It was an example of poor advance communications of delegates' needs by the conference organisers.

I think Wendy enjoyed attending her first international conference, and many delegates from outside the UK admired Caesar for being the perfect assistance dog. The conference lasted several days; she made many new contacts and subsequently became a regular attendee at international gatherings. To misquote Roy Strong's words 'it opened the windows of opportunity and led to the wide open fields beyond'.

Wendy had a new and important part to play in the assistance dog movement. She had next been invited to travel to London for a meeting about head injuries to discuss various cognition issues. There she met Princess Diana at St George's Hospital, who showed great interest in the circumstances of Wendy's accident. It was not surprising that some years after the tragic death of the Princess in 1997, when the Diana Memorial in Kensington Gardens was opened in July 2004, Wendy decided she would like to pay a visit. Access issues for dogs were just being considered in Government, since some dogs had been denied entry to taxis and other barriers had been created for them. When Wendy got to Kensington, she was turned away by the security staff at the memorial because Caesar was 'not a guide dog'. She had a similar experience when after obtaining tickets to watch tennis at Wimbledon, she was denied entry with her dog. She appeared in an interview on TV during an interval in the match play and spoke about how she had been told that the presence of a dog amongst the spectators might distract the players and was asked 'what about if the dog ran on the court to chase a tennis ball?'

With another door about to open, Wendy contacted her local Member of Parliament, Annette Brook about the access to the Diana Memorial, which had been built with public funds. The MP had been elected in 2001 and was made the Liberal Democrat spokeswoman for Home Affairs. Immediately she asked Wendy for more details, including photos of the signage 'Guide Dogs Only', and she brought the matter up in the House of Commons during question time. Later, when a meeting was arranged in Portcullis House, Westminster, to show how guide dogs differed from other assistance dogs, Wendy was one of the invited speakers. The guide dog owners and their representatives present seemed more concerned that the new office block for MPs had been opened with a main entrance that had clear glass doors and no symbols that would stop a blind person without a dog trying to walk through into the strong glass. Clearly people in wheelchairs had different needs from those who had visual disabilities, including blindness.

Wendy was invited to join various access committees. Caesar had actually been trained with the help of money donated by the Dutch-based Rabobank, and the Netherlands was another country where access was important. Peter Gorbing was able to advance Wendy's cause, which was taken up at the Royal Welsh Show, where the Kennel Club too became aware of dogs being kept out of places and gave their support. Caroline Taylor, then working from Banbury on publicity, arranged for photos of Caesar to go to the national press, to help overcome the objections to registered assistance dogs entering premises.

In 2005, Wendy was invited to fly to Croatia for the next IAHAIO Conference. There she was asked to research the European Countries that had passed disability access laws and those where there was no legal enforcement. Her research was published in an assistance dog journal later in 2005. Following this she was awarded a travel scholarship by International Assistance Dogs for Disabled People (IADDP), travelling with it in 2006 when she flew across the Atlantic with Caesar beside her, encouraged by the facilities offered by the airline. The flight took only six or seven hours, and Caesar travelled well and retained full control until arriving at the destination where toilet relief areas were found.

One of Wendy's problems when travelling through London had been that all the parks with grassed areas were locked at night, so it was difficult to find toilet areas for any dog travelling home in the evening. Some dogs even learnt to empty their bladders over the drains in the gutter, leaving no traces! When Wendy travelled she carried a 'little bag' for the dog, and the mystery of its contents, rather like a royal person's handbag, was revealed to me by Wendy. She carried a small teddy bear, a Nylabone to chew, a small blanket and little treats for rewarding him.

What else did the team of Wendy and Caesar achieve? On a local basis in 2004, she formed the Broadstone Access Group. After winning the scholarship in 2005 to go to the Assistance Dogs International (ADI) Conference, she gave the keynote speech on pet passports and dogs travelling from the USA to Europe.

This in turn lead to the holding of the 2008 international meeting of ADI in London, where for the first time several people came with their assistance dog from North America to attend a meeting held in Europe. When I arrived at the hotel near Heathrow airport, I was greeted by a call from a blind person whose dog was using the grass relief area outside the hotel; Ed Eames had recognized my voice from when I had spoken with him many years earlier at a USA service dogs meeting. Until then, their international conferences had always been held in North America. Wendy's travel experiences had encouraged partners with assistance dogs to visit the UK and Europe, with Peter Gorbing as President of ADI for the three-year term, so a truly international gathering at a hotel at Heathrow became possible.

In 2006, the Secretary of State for Transport invited Wendy to join the committee which was mainly dealing with access to public hire transport and especially taxis for people with disabilities. Until her involvement, most of the focus had been the needs of visually-impaired people, especially guide dog owners. She was next privately invited to advise the Metropolitan Police on certain disability issues. Wendy joined as a stakeholder to the group committee for the forthcoming 2012 Olympics; the organisation had representatives from many of the assistance dog groups. A number of assistance dogs, with their partners, were to be involved in carrying the Olympic Torch around Great Britain, but it fell to Wendy and Udo, the replacement for the retired Caesar, to advise the Olympic Committee and especially to show them the requirements of people travelling with assistance dogs to the various venues. Other items such as ticketing and the seating to allow room for a dog needed to be decided. Wheelchair ramps and toileting or 'relief areas' were to be available at all the venues for Olympic sports in 2012.

At the time of the previous Olympics, held in Beijing in the summer of 2008, Wendy had 'run' with the official torch on April 8th across London Bridge, of course accompanied by the willing Caesar escorting the torch whilst it was coming through London on the way to China. Apparently her skill had so impressed the Ambassador at the Chinese Embassy that Wendy was invited to go to view the opening Olympic ceremony there with many other guests. It was understood that this was the first time a dog had been allowed on the embassy premises, but Wendy was personally greeted on arrival by the lady Ambassador and all the staff there had been forewarned that the dog was 'friendly and very clean'.

Wendy said the embassy staff all had their eyes fixed on her, as she felt it must be an unusual sight for a dog to be moving among the other guests. Wendy told me she was able to sit next to Tessa Sanderson OBE, a javelin medallist (not usually throwing a discus though). Wendy had also been asked to advise on the clothing for the police who escorted the torch whilst it was taken round the country: in 2008 they had cyclists' uniforms but four years later when the torch went through every British county with police runners, they wore a more suitable grey uniform designed for their job.

Wendy attended nearly all the Assistance Dogs Europe (ADEu) annual meetings, flying with Caesar. Danny Vancoppermolle as ADEu

President asked her to promote the use of pet passports and microchip identification for all assistance dogs. Since 2004 the American based ADI had been negotiating with ADEu over standards so that there was equality and the two organizations were able to be brought together at Baltimore in 2007.

Peter Gorbing had retired as ADI President in 2012 after three years. At the Barcelona conference he received a standing ovation from all the delegates for the work he and his assistants had done in building a truly international organization that all could join on equal terms. Wendy had played a small but important part in involving international cooperation.

In 2006, Wendy had met Karen, who later had been trained with Coco as a medical alert dog. Wendy had suffered intermittent epileptic attacks following her head injury and within a year of getting Caesar she observed that he was able to indicate an approaching fit. Karen had been diagnosed with Addison's disease and when Caesar was in her presence, he started indicating for Karen an approaching Addisonian crisis. The condition, an immune disorder where the adrenal cortex fails to produce enough cortisol, is so sudden that collapse with hypoglycaemia will occur; it is an urgent condition and if undetected in advance, it means dialling 999 for an ambulance. A life-threatening condition.

Wendy already knew Claire Guest who had trained various medical alerting dogs, initially for epilepsy patients, diabetics etc. Claire was contacted by Karen and Wendy about having a dog specially trained for Addison's disease crisis detection and after a short delay Coco, a chocolate Labrador, was obtained. He was the seventh dog trained by Claire and has given valuable support to Karen, who travels a lot with Wendy, so the two dogs can play with each other happily.

In his tenth year Caesar was slowing up and was found to have anaemia. He had a haemangiosarcoma tumour causing an internal blood loss, but unfortunately it was not diagnosed immediately. After a marked deterioration one weekend he had to be rushed to a specialized veterinary centre where the scans showed spleen enlargement and a widely-spreading tumour. Even after a blood transfusion and an exploratory laparotomy, euthanasia became the only course of action. Caesar died in 2010. There then followed a 13-month period without an assistance dog, a most difficult time for Wendy, who suffered from the sudden bereavement and was not able to train for a replacement.

With the great success of Caesar as a Golden Retriever, Wendy specified that she wanted to stay with the same breed. Nearly all the dogs in training at Banbury were Labrador Retrievers or their first crosses. The selection of Golden Retrievers was a problem, as either their temperament or their health record was not right; even trying to breed Dogs for the Disabled's own Golden puppies had been a failure from the Golden brood bitch planned mating.

Sarah Brady had successfully trained Udo at Banbury kennels and Wendy came to stay there, accompanied by Karen as her carer and Coco as Karen's assistant dog. The training fortnight was conducted in the Frances Hay Centre. Qualifying on February 14th 2013, Udo soon took to the work of an assistance dog living in Dorset. Wendy now has the record of being the champion wheelchair geocacher, a pastime that gets you exploring out of doors using a GPS receiver, with the most 'finds' in the world. Wendy is the third highest of all the geocachers in England. Her hobby takes her to many countries where she can add to her total of finds'.

Wendy also made the national newspapers when a stray eagle flew into her sitting room early in 2014. The bird sat on her bookcase watching her until a bird rescuer arrived to catch the eagle and return it to its owner.

Wendy said recently to me: 'Disabled people living on benefits can't afford an assistance dog, the annual upkeep for a dog is growing every year'. The dog costs a client nothing throughout its training but then when home, the daily maintenance becomes a problem, and the climate for disabled people, Wendy thinks, has now become much harder. Looking at amputees, having a limb surgically removed cannot be compared with a man who has been blown up by a landmine, where there are big psychological issues; the quality of the skin is not the same as a young amputee's limb stump. After an injury you think back on how it might have happened and how it might have been avoided; after 20 years of pushing a wheelchair you end up with gnarled-up joints'.

Chapter 9

Canine Partners leads on; Dogs for the Disabled diversifies

In recent years, the parallel development of the two leading assistance dog charities has showed there could be benefits for the disabled in the range of services offered to clients in a more competitive situation. Diversification is defined as a strategy to grow a business; it involves taking a new product or service to a new group of customers with disabilities. Dogs for the Disabled had been the first charity able to move forward with a National Lottery grant to build its own centre at Banbury and become almost fully independent of the Guide Dogs for the Blind Association. The greater freedom allowed the charity to look at new areas where assistance dogs could be of help.

Canine Partners for Independence, based in Hampshire, were looking to train more assistance dogs in a new training facility, and a few years later they too received National Lottery funding. With additional funds they were able to plan a purpose-built centre in a rural area that had previously been used as a polo pony equestrian centre. Canine Partners for Independence became a registered charity in England & Wales in 1990. It then had to suffer a series of temporary homes, moving in 1994 from the front room of Anne Conway's house to other rented premises in Hampshire. For the next six years the charity leased premises in Hampshire, moving as the work of dog training expanded from Emsworth to Havant and to former chicken sheds at Petersfield. In 2001 the permanent site at Heyshott was purchased and building commenced. A National Lottery grant allowed for a forward-looking design to provide facilities for dogs and for residential classes.

The new Chief Executive, Alastair Lang, oversaw the work and a simplified title of 'Canine Partners' with a new purple livery was chosen. In 2000, 15 dogs had been placed which included the well-publicized Endal, who had won the Millennium award sponsored by Purina and Beta Foods and by the magazine *Dogs Today*. It was claimed that the dog could operate ATM cash machines and that one such dog could obey 154 identifiable commands.

With the centre's building activity taking place, only 12 dogs were trained, but there were many opportunities for publicity. Nina Bondarenko and Alan Parton were much involved in promoting the work of the charity; both of them I first met at Crufts, where they had a modest stand with a tombola wheel competition, I recall, but few dogs of theirs on show.

Canine Partners was relaunched in 2002 under the direction of Terry Knott as Chief Executive. A discussion with Dogs for the Disabled was set up in 2003 about closer cooperation between the two. Nothing came of it and Banbury for Dogs for the Disabled was producing far more dogs. It then took many years before an understanding was reached over areas to develop that were not conflicting the work of the two.

A satellite centre at Southampton had been set up by Canine Partners and they had been able to place ten dogs through the new centre in 2002. An invitation to become Canine Partners' Patron was made to the Duke of Gloucester following his visit to the new centre at

Heyshott. In 2003 Canine Partners said there were 77 working partnerships and the official recognition of the work of these assistance dogs was welcomed. Her Majesty the Queen received some of the dogs at a private demonstration behind closed doors at Windsor, and they made a good impression, but the event was not used in publicity.

Heyshott Training Centre was fully functional in 2005 and the official opening took place in the presence of the Patron, the Duke of Gloucester. More satellite centres at East Sussex, then at Hull, had been opened, which gave opportunities for clients and puppy socialisers (puppy parents) to meet and keep in touch with the Heyshott base. Endall was awarded 'Hero Dog of the Year' at Crufts that year. In 2002 Endall had reputedly saved the life of Alan Parton when he had fallen out of his wheelchair in a car park, and he became known worldwide as the 'Wonder Dog'.

Andy Cook, a very skilled assistance dog trainer with many years of experience with Hearing Dogs for Deaf Persons, was appointed as Director of Operations for Canine Partners and the charity was ready for a further step forward in its development. Nina Bondarenko became involved in a BBC TV documentary showing how disruptive teenagers might be brought into useful service by training dogs for assistance work. Her likeable personality came through, although the peak time TV show in April 2007 did not convince viewers that there was a good response amongst the young persons' group with only one apparent success. However it led Nina on to develop a lecture series which she gave round the country as well as in Australia in subsequent years, after leaving Canine Partners.

As dog training ability grew under Andy Cook, an appeal was made to build three purpose-built chalets suited for disabled people coming to be trained with dogs. The accommodation was opened in 2009; it allowed all training to take place at Heyshott rather than at off-site Holton Leed, Dorset. For the opening ceremony Baroness Margaret Thatcher came to Heyshott to cut the ribbon. With the retirement of Terry Knott that year, Andy Cook was promoted to Chief Executive Officer whilst keeping the Director of Operations role.

The years of recession after 2008 affected all charities' finances. 40 dogs were trained in 2008 and again in 2009 before confidence in the next decade allowed funding for an increase to 67 dogs by 2013. The annual reports show that the royal connections were maintained, with a visit by Prince Harry in 2010, a year when structural reorganization started following a 'stakeholder's consultation' the previous year. In readiness for an increase in the number of partnerships to be trained from 2011 and beyond, separate new posts were created: the Chief Executive, and a new appointment, Director of Operations.

Another innovation was a cooperative partnership with the charity Help for Heroes, who agreed to fund five canine partners trained with injured servicemen or women. Petty Officer Steve Brookes was the first person of many to benefit when he was matched with Major. More such assistance dog training followed, with the collaboration with the occupational therapy team at Headley Court (Ministry of Defence centre). By 2011, 44 new partnerships had been trained, and to meet the demand for dogs, a search was commenced for an additional training centre, and Fields Farm, near Loughborough Leicestershire was acquired with the necessary planning permission.

There were 110 puppies situated at satellite centres around the country, including Scotland, that were being prepared for their future work as assistant dogs in the years ahead. The purchase of the second centre was completed in January 2012 and a step-by-step plan to renovate the farm buildings was started as funds became available. Close to the M1, it could be used to start training dogs for more northern clients that year. 59 new partnerships were created in

2012 and 221 working partnerships were supported from one of three centres, with another 13 satellites for the puppy parents to attend were available.

The new Chairman of Canine Partners, Mark Richardson, took over in 2013. In that year 67 new partnerships were trained and 15 of these were trained at the new Midlands Centre as the building work there progressed. The charity was receiving 700 enquiries about dogs per year and the demand continued; the new centre was planned to provide 52 assistance dogs a year once the construction work was completed so the centre could be fully functional. Plans to increase number of assistance dogs each year were already showing results for Canine Partners to the benefit of their clients with disabilities on a waiting list for a dog.

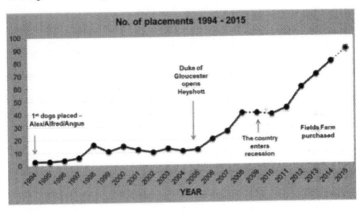

During the same period, Dogs for the Disabled had settled into the Banbury facility, which had the advantage of being close to modern shopping malls and supermarkets only a short drive away. It was necessary to have areas where dogs in training could be exposed to busy urban conditions, less than 10 minutes away from the rural setting of the kennels and offices. The need for improvements to the existing training hall and the expansion of kennel accommodation took up most of the available funds. After the Exeter guide dog kennels were closed in June 2002, it became important to provide a support centre in the south-west of England, where a number of clients were living.

Weston Super Mare seemed a suitable town, not far from the M5 with good road connections. A small industrial unit was converted to provide an office and a training room, but all dogs were housed off site in the homes of a number of volunteers. The supply of puppies to train was quite good and older dogs came from the GDBA. In 2003 there was an 80% training success, helped by the arrangement with the GDBA to receive dogs deemed unsuited for guide dog work. At a purchase cost of £2000 + VAT for these already well-trained assistance dogs, the price compared favourably with the price breeders were charging to buy an eight-week-old puppy.

The Dogs for the Disabled trustee board was strengthened with the addition of Mary Carden. A wheelchair user with experience in human resources management, she had been invited to join the trustee board in June 2002. She came in as a replacement for Jane McDonald, who had been the first Trustee appointed to represent the clients with dogs. Jane had extensive nursing experience and contributed frequently, but eventually, in March 2002, she felt it necessary to resign due to her ill health. She was elected as a Vice President in September. With her nursing connections she had appeared many times on TV with her dog, but her MS had progressed so that she could no longer travel to Banbury. It was possible to hold a final meeting of the training subcommittee in her home, in north London.

Following Jane's resignation it was decided that there should be room for two clients with assistance dogs, to serve on the board of Trustees. Andy Lee also joined the board with his experience of a uniformed officer who had suffered a disabling neck injury. There was a continuing number of enquiries from people asking for dogs, and the waiting time was then about eight months.

One of the main delays in the application process was in receiving a satisfactory medical report from the potential client's own medical practitioner. In the early years there were two medical doctors who successively volunteered for the trustee board to scrutinize applications, but it was impossible to find a third willing doctor, so reliance on outside medical reports became necessary. In some instances, a fee was paid by the charity for a doctor's report, but this did not necessarily mean a quicker reply.

I had attended an international meeting in Japan where a group of scientific workers produced a declaration at the 2005 conference in Tokyo of the International Association of Animal-Human Interaction Organisations (IAHAIO), encouraging all nations to give access to registered assistance dogs and stop any discrimination. In line with national policies, Dogs for the Disabled's Trustees had minuted in October 2001 that all references to 'handicapped' be removed from any communications.

Some time later, the Charity Commissioners visited Banbury. They were satisfied with our status and passed the charity's work and account keeping with only a few small recommendations. Of the two issues raised, one was over a Trustee who having done IT work for Dogs for the Disabled when his firm subsequently billed the charity fees unexpectedly, while another issue was related to whether insurance could be taken out to protect Trustees from claims in connection with their voluntary duties. The Trustees felt they needed protection, as all were volunteers and legal liabilities constrained their decisions. The commission eventually agreed to insurance being paid by the charity to reduce the risks.

Just before this, concerns were expressed amongst the Trustees over the activity of one board member who had made approaches to take over the chairmanship of the charity, he had the support of a single Trustee. He was involved in a local company that had offered

IT support for the charity through his firm, which many assumed was done on a pro bono basis. As events are still recent history, I do not name the individuals, although the dispute is based on the Trustee minutes kept at the time.

It came to a point when it required a vote of confidence to continue the charity on the existing basis rather than look to 'outsourcing' many of the activities. For the first time there was disharmony on the board, which later led to an apology and an offer of resignation. After the individual Trustee resigned in May 2002, the cost of software, which had proved unsatisfactory, had to be paid to the IT service company concerned, although the ex-Trustee had departed from the country. It was this payment that later caused a problem with the Charity Commission over a 'perceived Trustee benefit' through using the company he had been in charge of.

As difficulties had been created in the operation of the charity, I indicated at the next Annual General Meeting that it was time for a new Chairman to be selected. After 15 years helping the growth of Dogs for the Disabled with the help of many unpaid volunteers, I felt that there were new difficulties arising over budgeting and expenditure priorities at a time when I wanted to see more dogs trained to deal with the numerous applicants on the waiting list. The Trustees arranged to explore the situation with an 'away day' meeting arranged with an external facilitator attending to discuss all possible ways the charity should be developing. There was a good discussion on where the charity stood, but the emphasis was that more services to disabled people were to be developed. Inevitably a mission statement was to be written, as was now expected for all go-ahead organisations. Opportunities to sell training services to other bodies, looking for new areas to help people with disabilities and publicity to attract more donations all came up for discussion.

The recommendations were that a central services manager

should be appointed to look after the IT service needs and internal system support, while additional directors as key staff 'experts' were to be developed to provide specific programme support by 2003. The new chairman elected replaced me in February 2003. He had been fairly recently appointed as a Trustee but as well as living locally, he had management and financial skills suited to take on the Chairman's role.

The need to train more assistance dogs seemed then to take second place to increasing the number of fundraising staff to improve income. Ever since a 1998 report, emphasis had been put on developing fundraising groups, applying to charitable trusts, corporate partnerships with sponsorship and employee fundraising, public donations with links to clubs and societies and 'legacy marketing'. Much effort was to go into these developments over the coming years. New staff were hired; and one who saw the future as more charity shops soon left. Another proposed running raffles twice a year, but after a very good response to the first, subsequent mailings produced less money once costs were deducted.

A database of supporters from the earliest days had been built up; another proposal was to use the selling of dog training services to other groups. We had been successful in obtaining a major sponsor for the cost of the kennel rebuilding at Banbury and years later finding a donor for the complete sponsorship of the PAWS scheme to help parents and carers to have dogs helping autistic children. Once children's services were introduced, the legacy income grew spectacularly, particularly after the children with dogs featured in publicity. The income from wills and bequests developed well ahead of the Canine Partners income from this source when the published accounts were compared.

A further expansion of training to cover new areas was under consideration, as early in 1992 our client Gina Geary moved from South London to live in Scotland, where she had become the

'Honorary Scottish Representative of Dogs for the Disabled'. In 2009 the idea of a centre in Scotland was again put forward, but local funding was difficult to obtain and a previous application to the Scottish Lottery board in 2006 had been unsuccessful. The application made, for £100,000, was rejected on the grounds that there was no research to show that there was a need for training in Scotland. The Scottish Lottery Board suggested that Dogs for the Disabled could apply for the research funding on a possible need for training dogs in Scotland. No further progress was made there, since there had been difficulties in setting up research in 2006 when a previous researcher and supporter had moved away to the north west of Scotland and communication by her slow email was erratic. The trustees decided to concentrate on the northern counties of England; possible dog training sites were looked for in Yorkshire and Lancashire.

It was only many years later that funding was obtained from Scotland into looking at their local needs, with the Dementia Dog project. In 2013 it was reported that one in eight female deaths were caused by dementia, 2½ times higher than in 2003, according to national statistics There were opportunities for research into any benefits that assistance dogs could offer; younger dementia suffers and their spouses might be the group where a dog's presence in the home would give the greatest benefit.

The new chairman took over in 2003. He served successfully for several years until there was again a conflict over future management of the charity. One faction wanted to alter the executive's roles, but the majority of the board supported the Chief Executive's work. The Chairman tendered his resignation in April 2006, because, as he wrote, 'I can no longer be assured of the support of all the Trustees, which should I continue in office, would be to the detriment of the charity'.

I personally had got on well with my replacement as Chairperson, but there were organisational problems that arose which I had been barely aware of since I had moved away from the locality. Afterwards there were other Trustee resignations. Rosemary Smith, who had joined as Trustee in August 2003 and was experienced, having previously been the Chairperson at Canine Partners for many years, was persuaded to take on the Dogs for the Disabled Trustees' Chair. It was a temporary measure until a new person could be introduced to take on the increasingly important job.

The Trustees explored the training of dogs for children with special needs, and it was arranged that Helen McCain, as Training Director, should be asked to visit California to study how dogs were prepared for younger people there. In many charities' trust deeds, children were classed as aged from 11 to 25 years old. Jamie Sutherland had been injured in an accident when only 14: he was knocked off his cycle whilst delivering on a newspaper round, sustaining severe head injuries which would affect him for the rest of his life. When aged 16, he had trained with Kandy, and it was encouraging that he received the Pro Dog Pet of the Year award. Kandy worked as an assistance dog until she was 12, but then lived for a further four years with the family. Kandy was beside Jamie as he went through College and into his first job and later his marriage.

Two child partnerships were to be trained in 2004 as a pilot scheme; one boy's mother had already been to the States to see how children could benefit from assistance dogs, and she was well connected in the academic world and was instrumental in promoting a children's service. Her son, Percy, and a girl of a similar age, Kayleigh, were the first two children to get dogs in 2004, and the publicity at Crufts and elsewhere was very favourable. There were increased opportunities for fundraising to be applied in new areas, and the first royal visit to the centre by Princess Anne on April 2003 was another opportunity to show the increased range of disabilities that were being helped by assistance dogs. As the former Chairman of 15 years, I was pleased to be introduced to her again, as she was being conducted round the kennels by Peter Gorbing. She showed great interest in all the dogs and the work being done.

As a result of a special appeal to increase services, by October 2003 the large sum of £243,000 was received from Pets at Home for building and extending facilities in the kennels. Anthony Preston, the Chief Executive of the Pet Supermarket firm, continued to support the charity in various ways in the coming years and a valuable relationship was built up with the staff at their stores.

Improving the income remained a priority if further development of dog services was to take place. A successful bid to the BBC's Children in Need Appeal led to a grant to pay a dog trainer for three years to develop the service to provide dogs to children with special needs, and this proved to be successful in many ways. New ideas to use the trainers' skills and diversify the charity lead to the announcement of 'The Vision' in 2005. A new executive committee structure based on directors in several departments of the charity was started.

Dogs for Disabled's accreditation by Assistance Dogs International (ADI) was achieved in October 2005. ADI was a global organisation centred on North American programmes and giving a seal of approval of the work based at Banbury. The benefits of the vision were awaited; there were to be opportunities to train instructors from other countries at a fee and to develop advice and information services. The training of assistance dogs needed to increase, since only 25 qualifications were predicted in a year. Exeter, as a productive and reliable base, had been closed following a GDBA policy change and a replacement centre had taken some time to find. Sarah Brimblecombe wrote expressing her disappointment at the closure of the Exeter centre and offered to fund an aftercare visitor for clients in the south west of England. Some reorganisation for the south-west was necessary.

In 2004, after a change in the management structure, the fundraising strategy had been refocused, with greater emphasis on developing corporate opportunities. The proposal for a Legacy Officer, as used by large charities such as the RSPB, was put to one side, although this source of funding was subsequently to produce almost half the total income. There had been 331 qualifications to date, but it was only possible to prepare dogs for 32 adults and 12 children in 2006.

The standing of Dogs for the Disabled overseas led to Marta Czerwinska, whom I had met at a Warsaw Conference, applying in 2004 from Gdynia in Poland to study at Banbury; a lady from Germany also had previously come to the Ryton kennels to study, but then it was several years before a group from Spain came over to Banbury to study the work of training assistance dogs. Strong links were developed with Teo Mariscal of Bocalan, a charity founded in 1990, who worked with assistance dogs in Spain and in South America on AAT.

By 2006, the end-of-year accounts had a surplus of over £30,000 from an income of £1,460,471 and an expenditure £1,154,916. Events such as the sponsored 'Volcano challenge' had brought in £45,500; the previous year a Three Peaks Challenge had been started on this method for sponsored fundraising by 10 individuals, including the CEO. The name of the charity was attractive to people wanting to undertake sponsored events and to those making money bequests. In 2006, a legacy of £200,000 was the largest sum received out of a total of £537,969 raised through wills; the legacy income had increased once children and dogs were put together in the appeals. The reserves policy was for six months gross revenue expenditure for the year to be held, other funds went on expansion of the services.

In 2006, management issues were again brought to the notice of the Trustees following the resignation of a manager who had been at Banbury several years. Only 27 partnerships had been trained that year and a target of 40 dogs to be trained in 2007 would require more

DICK LANE

resources if the number of dogs trained was to increase. Developing new initiatives was taking up much staff time: prison pups, autism dogs, information services and again Scottish dogs were all under discussion. It was proposed that there was a need for a General Manager, a part-time Finance Manager and a Personal Assistant to the Directors. The Chief Executive would then concentrate on building external links with potential donors, increasing the profile of the charity through public affairs and communication, long-term planning and paving the way for new initiatives. Co-ordinating the new directors and ensuring managers were well focused, meeting issues and ensuring targets were met became part of the key role for the CEO.

Further recognition of the charity's work came in January 2007, when Peter Gorbing was elected as the President of Assistance Dogs International in Baltimore. It was the first time a person outside the USA had been honoured in this way; he handed over his European ADI Chair to Janet van Keulen. The number of new partnerships had been planned to increase up to 40 in the coming year, but maternity leave for trainers and instructors and some resignations were limiting the number of assistance dogs qualifying each year. Instructors were producing up to six dogs a year, insisting on the highest quality, but the productivity was lower than comparable organisations overseas where absence through maternity leave seemed to have less impact. The recruitment of more trainers was necessary, with a development business plan focused on a centre for Northern England as a physical base.

An information service for disabled people who wished to have a companion dog was another idea put forward in the three-year plan; 2007 was the final year of the BBC Children in Need three-year grant, and new areas of work for children were being looked at. An application to the Scottish Lottery for a centre there was again made unsuccessfully, as many funds were then being directed at the forthcoming Olympics. Rosemary Smith agreed to remain as

Chairperson after her first year in office but wished to continue only until the December. The new Chairman, John Starley, provided a safe pair of hands with a strong financial background and a practical approach to the work of producing assistance dogs. The recruiting of other Trustees with commercial backgrounds continued as new developments occurred.

In 2007 the supply of sufficient puppies for the puppy socialiser scheme was causing difficulties with increased numbers required, and it was decided to start breeding with bitches whelping in the dog carers' own homes. We had to look for more bitches to produce puppies, preferably those proven from the GDBA Breeding Centre's lines. The breeding scheme was set up using Labrador females, as Golden Retrievers were harder to find as brood bitches. There were only 56 puppies out on the scheme, 10 adult dogs were in advanced training and three dogs were in training for ASD children.

The proposal from Helen McCain, as Training Director, had been to have enough brood bitches to provide 30% of the annual puppy supply requirement. It was something I had suggested years earlier soon after the move to our own kennels at Banbury, but the idea was not taken up at that time because of a lack of experienced people. A continuing difficult was to find Golden Retriever females of the standard needed for training, and this led to delays in providing replacement dogs for those clients who specified that breed or a first cross with a Labrador.

In May 2008, a permanent base for training in Yorkshire was found at Nostell Priory near Wakefield, a successful facility from which courses could be run was opened under Louise Hart's leadership. She had been working from her Yorkshire home since 2002 and was joined by a second instructor in 2003. Partly-trained dogs were sent up from Banbury and the two instructors were able to produce many successful partnerships in the north of England.

Lisa Dixon was a client who had applied to Dogs for the Disabled when her son Thomas was only two, even before Nostell opened. She had to wait until he was six before she was able to attend Nostell for a week to get Vito, a lively pale-coloured Cocker Spaniel. Vito was a great success, walking steadily beside Thomas' walking frame. Thomas used to avoid any eye contact, but his mother said how he enjoyed talking to others and attends secondary school with the dog ready to greet him daily as he comes out of school at the end of the afternoon. As described in her interview, the 'companionship, unconditional love, physical contact and Vito staying in reach so Thomas could stroke and talk to him' were greatly beneficial in providing social support for him.

In 2009 some 25 adults and 18 children were trained as the total of 43 for the year, compared to 39 the previous year but we hoped for 56 dogs if the target was reached. There next came out a 10-year plan which provided for 275 puppies on the socialising scheme and 180 dogs qualified by 2020. The 2012 five-year plan was that by 2017, training would be aimed at reaching 47 assistance dogs for adults and 18 assistance dogs for children with disabilities in addition an increase to 33 dogs for autism assistance, totalling 98 in a year.

There was a need too for more training centres, which led to a move from Weston to Bristol with better facilities. In addition to the existing Yorkshire base at Nostell, a new centre was opened in Lancashire. The use of part of the kennel premises at Atherton, where there was a purpose built GDBA centre, was made possible by 2013. New sources of income in 2015 enabled Dogs for the Disabled to state, 'These improvements will make the charity better equipped to meet its target of training 98 dogs per year by 2018, almost doubling its current output'.

The demand for assistance dogs for young people led to setting up the PAWS service as a new initiative in 2010. It was fortunate that in December of that year, Dogs for the Disabled was nominated as one of the three Christmas charities of the *Daily Telegraph*. Work on the new PAWS project was developing well and opening up new contacts, once it was given the confidence of a three-year sponsorship by a single benefactor. Some of the new services could bring in additional resources to support general running costs, the Chief Executive stated, and the 2011 priority was thus to maximize the opportunities of the PAWS project and to support the development of it in other countries, especially Australia, where the PAWS sponsor, Mel Gottlieb, through the RSI Trust donor was based.

Stitchting Helphunds took up the PAWS idea in the Netherlands, but the Royal Guide Dog School subsequently became the PAWS developers for that country. New income streams required more staff, but some projects generated income, such as the work for the Kingswood Trust which specialized in providing supported living for adults with autism, largely funded from grants from local authorities. In return for statutory support service, they were sufficient to pay for a dog trainer's attendance.

Since 2004, a USA-published report showed that canine visitors acting as therapy dogs had benefits for young children's learning and wellbeing in classrooms and hospitals. 'Learning Companions' was another area that could cooperate with Dogs for the Disabled's skill with dogs; two dogs could become therapy dogs, leading to further opportunities for animal assisted interventions (AAI). The use of dogs as adjuncts to therapy with various special needs was growing in Europe, and AAI would expand the work of assistance dogs; 'activity dogs' required far less training input. Dogs for the Disabled planned for a modest increase to 48 dogs trained in 2012 for the established adults' assistance dog production; it was decided at the Trustee meeting held at the same time to explore and develop new uses for assistance dogs. Animal assisted therapy (AAT) had been carried out in many countries and was recommended, since it would allow dogs to be usefully employed even though they were unsuited for the adults' regular training scheme.

The proposed 'development of innovative services that are life-changing for our clients' was requiring a diversification into new areas where dogs could help. An Armed Services project was not developed, since Canine Companions were better able to reach Headley Court in the south and even the rehabilitation centre at Catterick in Yorkshire. Later the new charity Hounds for Heroes started to obtain a lot of publicity and collected funds that left less room to start up a specific facility by Dogs for the Disabled.

Neurological conditions such as post-traumatic stress disorder (PTSD) were an area where dogs might assist: it was being explored in Oxford, linked to Banbury centre, as another development for AAI therapy dogs. In 2012 the Social Enterprise development was considered further. John Pepin conducted a feasibility study as a consultant from Aperio group. New areas of diversity were considered by the Trustees: therapy dogs, rehabilitation dogs, the training of security or guard dogs, autistic spectrum disorder assistance dogs, community and geriatrics therapy dogs were all development opportunities. Dogs trained to sniff out bed bugs as a service to hotels and guest houses was another suggestion similar to the one operated in the Medical Detection Dogs scheme. Vine mealybug detection dogs had been used in the vineyards in California by Bonita Bergin, and there could be openings to detect other invasive insect pests in the UK, using dogs' highly-developed scent discrimination.

Fungal tree diseases could be another area to train dogs in detection of infection by scenting. A plan for the five years 2011 to 2015 in the published Annual Report outlined the direction the charity wished to take. It stated: 'Dogs for the Disabled is a small innovative charity that recognizes the extensive capacity for dogs to help disabled people in a wide range of ways. We are seeking to increase the output of assistance dog partnerships by 45% during the life of the plan. At the same time, the charity will seek to touch the lives of many more disabled people and their families by developing services that enable them to fulfil their lives through interactions with a trained dog. Collaborating with other charity and not-for-profit partners where possible, we seek to use our expertise to encourage the developments'. The same report also noted that during 2013, two longstanding Trustees had retired: 'Rosemary Smith and Dick Lane both had chaired the Board of Trustees in the past and brought enormous skills, experience and energy to the charity'.

In 2014 Dogs for the Disabled trained 51 assistance dogs and 110 families obtained dogs through the PAWS scheme, bring the total of families who had benefited from the three day training and information scheme to get a dog to 600.

Chapter 10

Some of the science in the use of assistance dogs

Attachment is a frequently used word when speaking about dog partnerships, and it has largely replaced the human-animal bond (HAB) spoken and written about previously. This chapter looks at some recent knowledge of the interaction of people and animals; it combines and links current knowledge from psychology, behavioural biology, psychophysiology and endocrinology. Humans and companion animal species share many common features due to evolutionary history and convergent selection; maternal behaviour and bonding between mother and infant occurs in all our species. Dogs share with other mammals structures and functions of the brain, and much canine behaviour and other activities are those common to the original wolf-type animal.

An evolutionary approach to dog domestication is that 'hunter gatherers', with their children and women in their dwelling places, were likely to have been the first to take in orphaned cubs and rear them as companions before releasing them back into the 'wild'. There is a natural response for all females to nurture helpless and soft newborn creatures, and puppies kept with nomadic people fall into this group. Progressive selection of wolf-type animals that became more accustomed to being closer to people led to choosing to keep those that would eventually live closer to the dwelling places, and once there, they would rely more on scavenging. Food scraps were thrown to them, especially at times when there was more meat to eat than necessary for human survival. Women too have a predilection for looking after young animals and this was considered a favoured feature in people as a good predictor of being able to look after babies born in the future. Rearing puppies close to dwellings would have been encouraged, and domestication followed these close contacts.

Possibly around one hundred thousand years ago, our human species was developing general intelligence and becoming good at dealing with changes in food supplies and the climate. They were able to predict food scarcity and would migrate to areas where food was obtainable. In contrast the Neanderthal species was more powerful, but when climate cooling took place they were unable to adapt to the environmental changes; even with a hairy coat they did not survive the extreme cold as the ice sheets moved over northern Europe and beyond. It also seems possible that those canines more used to following nomadic humans would also have had a better chance of coming through periods of extreme cold.

Later animals became used as additional 'tools' to help the human hunters. At first the canines behaved as camp followers whose only function was to scavenge waste and raise the alarm by howling when predators were about. Dogs could run faster than spear-carrying men and by chasing they could exhaust a hunted animal, making it easy for the hunters to bring down at the end of the chase. A bond would develop with a hunting dog that helped to obtain meat more easily.

The behaviours of wolves and dogs has been extensively studied. Behaviours of dogs compared to that of wolves have been debated for many years, based on a hierarchical pack system that was once thought to typify the social behaviour of the wolf. Some false conclusions were drawn when small groups of wolves kept in zoo-type enclosures were observed by researchers. Dog trainers took up the idea of looking for direct links with wolves and the need for a dominant figure in the pack, even when the pack consist only of the owner and the dog. Punishment had been seen to occur naturally when a bitch growled at her puppies or pushed them away for sucking at her too painfully.

The idea that the wolf pack was in continuous conflict encouraged trainers to use punishment to eliminate an undesired behaviour. It was wrongly assumed that punishment reduced the dog's status in the pack, even when man became the pack leader. The mistakes had been made when focusing too much on dominance, as had been seen from when wolves were watched in semi-captivity. Until continuous video recording was possible, the rather more difficult task of watching free-roaming packs of wolves had given strange ideas about pack behaviour.

Canada and Russia are two countries where it has been possible for patient observers to follow the interaction of groups of wolves in different packs. Tracking pack movements and video monitoring of behaviours showed a totally different set of relationships from those seen in captive wolf groups. Dominance in the wild was not observed by a single pack member; rather there was a rotation of the lead role in the group, depending on the challenges faced. There was a more comfortable relationship in the free living wolves based on family groups, often with the oldest bitch as the leader. Hunting packs worked as a group but without one dominant leader.

Painted or African Wild Dogs (*Lycaon pictus*), also known as Cape Dogs in South Africa, have a similar harmonious existence within the group. Packs I have observed had divided up for hunting, yet on return to the group, there was much nuzzling and interaction of one pack member with another. In two African groups I watched, one member had a twisted hind limb from a previous leg fracture, yet it would greet others and be greeted back as an equal, even though it was obviously disadvantaged as a hunter. The same cooperating behaviour is not seen in packs of scavenging or feral dogs that feed on rubbish heaps on the edges of towns, which do not behave like wild canids with wolf-type social groups.

Much of the behaviour of the domestic dog has evolved away from wolves and is the result of living with or near to people and the need to survive in times of famine or flood, adapting themselves to a niche close to human needs.

Another advance was to study the genetic relationship of the domestic dog to the free living wolf. Researchers analysed mitochondrial DNA from 162 wolves at 27 localities worldwide and from 140 domestic dogs representing 67 recognised breeds. This research supported the theory that wolves were the ancestors of dogs. Sequences from both dogs and wolves showed considerable diversity. The sequence divergence suggested that dogs originated more than 100,000 years ago, but the relationship was close enough for wolves to occasionally breed with dogs; other wolf lineages indicated episodes of admixture between wolves and dogs. Repeated genetic exchange between dog and wolf populations may have been an important source of variation for artificial selection. Most dog sequences belonged to a divergent branch and its descendants (the clade) but shared no sequences with wolves within this dog clade.

Konrad Lorenz, the Austrian who founded the science of ethology and initiated animal behaviour studies, thought that jackals were the ancestors of the non-northern breeds of dogs and the remainder had developed from wolves. In 1999 DNA studies proved him wrong; in fact the separation of a primitive wolf type from the primitive dog type took place thousands of years earlier than he thought. Behaviour studies were also unfortunately influenced by the wild-bred silver foxes kept for fur farming, where domestication took place in only 40 cage-bred generations: 10% selected for tameness in each generation were progressively bred with others selected for the same traits.

Most dog breeds have only developed in the last 250 years based on selection for a particular 'show' characteristic, but breeding from closed blood lines has produced more single gene disorders and complex ones as well. Before the development of specimen show dogs (the first national dog shows were in the 1860s), dogs were only selectively bred for function. Good scent and sight hunters, fast game chasers as well as attentive and alert protection of humans were chosen. Some of these breeds now form the most reliable stock for training as assistance dogs. Where good scenting is required, as for medical detection dogs, it is among the working game-retrieving breeds where the best results are obtained. They work for long periods and seem to enjoy the scent detection duty

Animals were developed as companions even when they were no longer needed in hunting or guarding. The relationship arose through the dogs' closeness to people, perhaps in communities after gathering in crops by harvesting or securing sources for other food supplies. In consequence of this evolutionary process, empathy towards animals and domestication of food species grew as people became more settled in their living places. The food crops could be grown once communities of people settled in a location where they had a regular supply of moisture for crops and water to drink. A more settled existence allowed for group interactions, with emotional bonds or attachment between persons outside the family or even to develop semi-domesticated animals, as farming the land became possible.

The theory of the attachment mechanism between mother and

child was developed in the last century by American psychologists and has since been extended to companion animals. Psychologist John Bowlby in 1969 was the first attachment theorist, describing attachment as a 'lasting psychological connectedness between human beings'. He believed that the earliest bonds formed by children with their caregivers have a tremendous impact that continues throughout life. Mothers who are available and responsive to their infants' needs establish a sense of security. The infant knows that the caregiver is dependable, which creates a secure base from which the child can explore the world. Brain activity for speech develops months before babies speak their first word, but a puppy's ability to communicate develops far more slowly and is limited. Visual cues are appreciated by both babies and puppies early in life, which allows a form of understanding between the parents or the siblings. The domesticated dog develops as a similar attachment figure for caring men and women, providing through contact and its activities a sensitive and socialising stimulation. Such an attachment is made easier by the number of dog breeds and variations; you can choose a strong, positive dog, a soft fluffy dog or one with a flattened baby-like face.

It has been suggested that humans have a basic need for closeness to animals. Prehistoric prey and predator relationships helped in finding greater security, in which dogs and humans gained benefits from each other's presence. The biophilia idea of humans needing natural contact with living plants and animals has since been developed to explain why people feel more relaxed when animals are around them. Some disorders in human health are now attributed to a 'nature deficit' problem; it is claimed certain illnesses can be reduced by exposing individuals to a type of nature therapy often involving animals.

The attachment of children to dogs and other small animals is well recognised. Attachment theory provides a biopsychological concept that allows the integration of these psychophysiological, behavioural and endocrinological research findings. Attachment is a behavioural system that ensures that the child maintains or establishes proximity to the attachment figure, particularly when the child is stressed or in danger. This ultimately serves in the protection of the children; it is important for attachment but there is a need to have a bond with an animal before such support can happen.

Dr Andre Beetz from Rostock reviewed the latest research as well as used her own data when she spoke at the Assistance Dogs International conference in London, presenting an 'interdisciplinary, integrative model of human-animal relationships'. She said children who were exposed to parental neglect, abuse or inconsistent behaviour formed an insecure attachment which interfered with the effective regulation of stress and anxiety and with the ability to develop trustful relationships later in life. Since attachment patterns are generally transferred to other caregivers, these children are unable to accept social support from caregivers to the same extent as securely attached children. However, these same children may engage in close and trusting relationships with pets, suggesting that insecure attachment patterns are not transferred to pets. Thus, relationships with animals may have a great potential to break the cycle of transmission and to promote regulation of stress and anxiety. Also in insecurely-attached children, the hormone oxytocin may be released by petting and interaction with the pet. If a child develops a secure relationship with an animal in a pedagogical or therapeutic setting, it might also be easier for a teacher or therapist to establish a secure relationship with the child. When there were insecure attachment patterns that children had developed with their parents, normally an attachment might then get re-established in the children's relationships with professional caregivers, such as teachers or therapists.

The results support the hypothesis that relationships with animals may have a great potential to break the transmission of insecure attachment. If a child develops a secure relationship with an assistance animal, it might also be easier for a teacher or therapist to establish a secure relationship with the child. Dr Beetz's research showed that during periods of anxiety, the lowest cortisol levels were found in children with a real dog compared to a stuffed toy dog. Among the children with insecure/disorganized attachment, the data suggest that children with insecure attachments became calmer and could tolerate stress better when a live dog was present. Similar results were found in research reported in Austria. The more a child stroked and talked to the dog, the lower his or her cortisol, and a dog supported the children in coping with social stress more efficiently than a human. Not all children are the same however; children differed in their ability to benefit. The more actively the child related to the dog, the greater the stress-dampening effect in children aged between four and 12 years old in this research.

'One Health' research on attachment theory was also conducted by Dr June McNicholas at the University of Warwick with her colleagues in the 1990s, and she was also able to work closely with the clients of Dogs for the Disabled. I presented her research, as one of her two co-authors, at an international conference in Japan in 1995. I was able to give a good account of what Dogs for the Disabled had achieved in England. Further work on attachment by June with G M Collis at the same university is frequently quoted in publications as a source of information on assistance dog benefits. Having an assistance dog will require the individual to take more exercise and provide more exposure to the outdoors and natural ecosystems, since the dog will require two or more walks a day. The dog's closeness to nature in town parks or on country walks introduces the client as well as the dog to the new sights, colours and smells of the out-of-doors environment. Benefits to the client and dog are modulated through the nervous and immune systems.

The 'One Health' approach is now more widely recognised as playing a part in Animal Assisted Interventions (AAI), since institutional life is no longer considered obligatory for those with special needs. More research on attachment was being conducted in many countries into dog and human relationships: the USA, Germany, Austria and Italy. The study by Andrea Beetz in Germany had been conducted on a large group of 162 at-risk children where their attachment was disturbed. Where a child developed a secure relationship with an animal assisting in the home or at school it was easier for a teacher or therapist to establish a secure relationship with the child.

Recently, research at Sussex University by Victoria Ratcliffe and Attila Andics looked at the effects of different types of human speech on the dog's brain. They found dogs were paying attention to emotion and information from the person speaking as well as understanding the actual words. This explains the large range of words that assistance dog owners have found their dogs respond to and builds up the emotional bond that helps to overcome loneliness.

Insecure human and animal attachments

With the increasing use of dogs to help children with special needs to develop their full potential, more work needs to be done on the ways the dogs are helping. The anecdotal evidence is now strong, but the mechanisms, such as those of communicating with severely autistic children, are still not fully understood. The transmission of attachment patterns from one attachment relation to another is a standard in human-human relationships. Hence insecure attachment patterns that children have developed with their parents normally get re-established in the children's relationships with the professional caregivers, such as teachers or therapists. An experienced dog trainer can obtain the trust of the child, who in turn will become able to trust the assistance dog. This is especially tragic for those children who may already have developed a disorganized attachment, since this pattern can jeopardise their further development. Matching a dog becomes less easy with such a child and the skill of the instructor is important.

Researchers Janelle Nimer and Brad Lundhal looked at all the published reports on Animal Assisted Therapy (AAT) in 2007 and concluded that young children were more accepting of animals' influences. AAT was as effective as other interventions or more; young children consistently benefited from all the outcome variables, including symptoms associated with autism.

Some of the hormones known to be involved in forming attachments and determining behaviours

Neurochemicals are produced within the body and are responsible for producing longer-lasting effects than those responses resulting from nerve stimulation. The prick of a needle produces a rapid response with a cry or a snatch away of the injured part; the pain may be quickly over but with most hormones once secreted they will alter the mood or the body's reaction for days or weeks. These neurochemical secretions seem able to alter people's brains in ways that help them to form caring, long term relationships with a new child. The increased secretion or 'surges' of the hormones oxytocin and prolactin at the time of childbirth are well known in women, but they are also linked to particular physical processes. Oxytocin is known best for its stimulation of muscular contractions during birth, but it has other wider effects. Prolactin promotes lactation, and the two together are thought to help in bonding the mother psychologically with her baby.

A rise in oxytocin levels has also been found in fathers at the time their spouse gives birth, which lead to the conclusion that interactions of close contact with the newborn triggers the neuro-hormonal system that underlies bond formation in humans. Oxytocin secretion is also known to rise in response to elevated levels of stress, so that might be part of an explanation of the father's reaction during birth, as was suggested by Dr Craig of Kings College Institute of Psychiatry.

Recent research on the role of oxytocin in social bonding in dogs extended the idea that it helps in the formation of relationships. First it is necessary to understand where other hormones are affecting moods and behaviours, also in insecurely attached children where oxytocin may be released by petting and interaction with the pet.

Cortisol is one of several hormones produced in the adrenal gland and it has the function of taking over and maintaining the body state if a flush of adrenaline from the same glands has fairly quickly worn off. Adrenaline stimulation is now commonly recognised by people who have been frightened or have to undergo some activity of the 'chase or frolic' type. Rapid breathing, a raised pulse rate and mouth dryness are some of the signs indicating adrenaline release. The hormone group known as corticosteroids, which includes cortisol, has effects on almost every organ of the body. Cortisol plays an important role in maintaining the tone of blood vessels and the regulation of fluid moving in and out of the circulation. A rise in levels of cortisol is found as a most important response to stress, severe illness, trauma and infections. It is the response involving cortisol in stressful situations that is of most interest to animal behaviourists. Acute stress can be considered a good response: it is adaptive and allows the body to return to a normal state as the cortisol level diminishes. Where a dog remains under stress due to some continuing problem, cortisol and ß endorphins remain at a high level in the blood, the dog becomes less reliable and unpredictable behaviours may result. There is now an increased awareness of the long-term effects of raised cortisol levels. Measuring cortisol has become possible by taking saliva or blood samples for analysis to also include IgA, Reactive Oxygen Metabolites (D-roms) and Biological Antioxidant Potential (BAP). All have been used in the assessment of stress in working dogs.

Oxytocin is one of nature's signalling systems, particularly relevant to the development of animal attachments. The hormone has the same chemical structure in all animals and as found in humans: it is a 9 amino acid long polypeptide, which means is not possible to give it by mouth, as it is destroyed by digestion. Oxytocin is produced in the brain from the part known as the hypothalamus, more specifically in the paraventricular and supraoptic nuclei of the pituitary. The neurons in the brain may act by influencing the activity of other signalling systems; serotonin and dopamine are secreted whilst others transmit opiodergic, cholinergic, and noradrenergic messages. Oxytocin was often used as an injection by farm vets as an effective medication during and after the birth of the young. In humans, spraying a solution up the nose is another method used to apply oxytocin in the study of hormone response and reactions. Experimentally it was possible to give oxytocin this way without the need to inject the patient every time. Once the neurons that connect with important regulatory areas of the brain are stimulated, the release of oxytocin from the hypothalamus into the circulation takes place, where it exerts a multitude of effects. The best-known response, easily demonstrated by the farm vets, was the stimulation of the muscles of the uterus and it was also used for the almost immediate 'let down' of milk from the mammary glands. After an injection of oxytocin it either caused contractions for a more rapid birth or in the suckling animal a gush of milk from the teats. When used this way, the therapeutic response was good but the effects lasted for only brief periods. It was even used in reptiles to help expel eggs, but was considered too painful to use in birds when they were 'egg bound'.

In recent years it has been realised that on the release of oxytocin from the brain, it acts against cortisol and reduces anxiety, with a calming effect. Oxytocin can produce an increase in the trust of others, encouraging interactive behaviours of several kinds.

The wider and more recently-discovered actions of oxytocin are of importance to those working with or using assistance dogs. Making friends, trusting and bonding may all be stimulated, while at the same time oxytocin induces a feeling of wellbeing, including the stimulation of social interaction and health promotion as well as a reduction in stress. Experimentally, a heightened awareness has been described after oxytocin is applied as a spray into the human nose, and the ability to interpret social cues is enhanced as all the senses' response is heightened. The mechanism of oxytocin is not fully understood, but the hypothalamus pituitary axis (HPA) activity decreases and the sympathetic nervous system is inhibited, leading to a lowering of blood pressure. The level of pain and inflammation when oxytocin is present may be reduced; oxytocin also stimulates the anabolic metabolism and thus has restorative properties.

The releasers of oxytocin may be found in many inter-animal contacts. After birth takes place and during the feeding process, the newborn stimulates nerve endings in the skin of the mammary glands. At the time of mother and baby interaction before breast feeding, oxytocin is released with fluid soon appearing at the nipples. In addition any skin contact, touch, light pressure, body warmth or stroking will activate the same nerves in the skin and stimulate the pituitary in the brain to produce oxytocin at a low level. Even more recently it has been shown that the skin of the chest and the abdomen also has the sensory nerves that respond by stimulating the pituitary and this had been applied when fathers of newborn babies are involved in nurturing and the pressing of their bodies together.

Oxytocin levels were shown to increase in these males, and this would account for the stronger relationships found between some fathers and their offspring. The importance of this observation is that the same response would apply when other forms of skin stimulation, such as that from contact with animals, release oxytocin, helping in the so-called 'bonding' of the two subjects. Elsewhere, using the face to face 'body hug' was instrumental in the bonding of relationships amongst primates, and it can be applied by parents for similar responses for oxytocin release; such contacts were considered important in developing affectionate relationships. This effect was first demonstrated in laboratory rats, where cortisol and oxytocin could be measured even whilst they were asleep. Pinching the toe of a sleeping rat caused a rise in cortisol as a response to pain, but stroking the rat on its abdomen with a soft toothbrush reduced the cortisol level since more oxytocin was released. Conscious rats stroked on the fronts of their bodies reacted similarly. This response was compared to the effect when a baby placed on the mother's breast skin was producing a similar release of oxytocin. This theory can be applied to the benefit of children being able to touch the bodies of animals.

Social bonding between people may involve a low-level oxytocin response; it may occur in people where a negative reaction to a relative stranger may be replaced by warmer feelings. An animal close to a human, such as a dog or a cat or even a horse, may serve as a releaser of oxytocin, especially when the animal is touched or stroked.

It was shown in Sweden that seriously-affected autistic children will respond to a horse nuzzling them when the child was left sitting on the ground. After an interval, the child allowed itself to be lifted up and start touching the horse with greater interactions than any previous attempts to make contacts with the apparently socially-isolated child. Some dogs by their very presence seem to have the ability to release oxytocin in humans, and such dogs when studied have been shown to produce more social interaction, to reduce anxiety and to increase trust. Cortisol levels measured in one experiment were seen to reduce blood pressure, after interaction with a dog coming into a room. Such results help to explain the health-promoting effect of having a dog, or any another animal.

The research study with June McNicholas in 1995, where about one hundred owners of assistance dogs trained by Dogs for the Disabled were interviewed, also showed that there were distinct health benefits. Questionnaires were sent out and a proportion whom I interviewed, as well as many phone contacts, were analysed by June and showed a positive human health benefit.

It was at that time not possible to fully explain why 47% of those persons with disabilities interviewed said their health had actually improved since receiving an assistance dog. It is suggested now that attachment to a dog is important for human health through its influence on the neuroendocrine mechanisms that can develop in human animal interactions. Other factors, such as more exercise and the dog's presence bringing in more opportunities to talk to people, would also contribute to perceived improved health.

Dogs too can benefit from their associations with people. The human-animal interactions described are important for human health, but it was also found by researchers that oxytocin levels in dogs respond to having close contact with humans. The early socialisation of puppies and human contact from two weeks of age onwards produces a dog which is easier to train later; the benefits seen were combined with a removal of punishment in training routines.

These facts were confirmed in Sweden, where Linda Handlin reviewed the relationship of cortisol and oxytocin hormones in the rapport between dog owners and their dogs. She set out to observe ten middle-aged ladies who owned Labradors, watching reactions over the period of one hour. Each subject was asked to spend three minutes petting, stroking and talking to their dog at the beginning of the experiment; this was followed by collecting seven serial blood samples from each person and from each dog to measure oxytocin and cortisol levels. The dogs' blood samples showed a significant rise in oxytocin after the first three minute; cortisol levels rose after 30 minutes in the dogs but their heart rates became lower during the hour of measurement. Heart rate was lowered in the women, but it was not possible to show any real change in their hormone levels. The conclusion was that short-term periods of stroking the dog and a sensory interaction between the dog and the human influenced hormone levels and lowered heart rates.

In the Swedish study with the ten Labradors, oxytocin was found to have a close relationship with the formation of bonding and attachment as well as its stress-reducing effect. Dogs that were kissed every day by their owners had higher oxytocin levels, as did their owners.

The age group of ladies studied may not necessarily apply to other groups of people with dogs and the results could not be extended to all dog owners. More research is called for, especially in dogs with disability groups, but oxytocin has repeatedly linked with dog attachment and social support. Previously, in the 1980s, the long-term health benefits seen over 10 years with protection against strokes were reported by studies of patients in the USA by Friedman and subsequent researchers. The personality and owners' need for attachment was examined by Manuela Wedl, a researcher from the University of Vienna, who said that dogs' attachment to their human partners was strongly affected by the closeness of the dog to the sitting owner. When the dog-regulated distance was increased, the dog personality axis of 'vocal and aggressive behaviour' was negatively related to this parameter.

When recognising 'neuroticism' in owners, the dog's attachment to its owner was strongly affected by its own personality. The more the owner thought of the dog as a social supporter and an understanding partner, the more often the dog came close to the owner. Observations were made where there were two dogs in the home, especially to look for the continuation of close, non-sexual bonding between dogs. The dogs' responses were studied in a research project published in 2014.

Pairs of dogs from the same household were chosen and one placed in an empty room in the presence of the familiar owner but not touched nor spoken to, and its activity was observed. Half the dogs were given oxytocin sprayed into the nose and the other half, as the control group, had a saline spray for the nose. When the second dog of each pair was brought in as well, the two dogs were watched for the next hour. The repeated video observations showed that the dogs that had the oxytocin tried to interact with their owners much more than those in the control group; they also tried to interact with the control group dogs who were less interested in making contacts. The oxytocin seemed to make the treated dogs more willing to greet other dogs and also attach to their human partners.

This confirms the benefits of stroking and grooming dogs when setting out to establish a firm bond between the assistance dog and the child or adult receiving and keeping the dog. Oxytocin is readily released by closeness and touch; the hormone is released in the brain where it exerts anxiolytic effects and decreases the activity in the HPA axis and in the sympathetic nervous system. As skin contacts are important to release oxytocin, the suggestion had been made that as massage of the shoulders was being used to reduce aggression of children in special needs schools, oxytocin nasal sprays might also have a beneficial effect.

There may be a reluctance of carers and teachers to get too close to their 'difficult' children. Dogs could play an important role in such situations and encouraging reports on the use of 'School Dogs' have come in as anecdotal evidence.

Testosterone

The effects of excess male hormone does not cause real problems to assistance dogs since nearly every dog trained has been neutered (castrated), usually at about six months of age. In the past testosterone was blamed for dominance and aggression in male dogs and castration was frequently advised for dogs that became too difficult for trainers to work with. Socialisation and reward-based training has gone a long way to showing that testosterone is not necessarily harmful in male dogs if they are handled correctly. Allowing attachment between dog and human to develop from an early age and avoiding unpredictable requirements from the dog can produce a calm and satisfactory companion in a dog. It may to some extent decrease the need for drugs or simply create a more positive calm and rewarding friendship in a health-promoting situation for those with special needs.

There had been rare exceptions to my knowledge where a man would ask to train with an 'entire' guide dog, often based on a previous experience with a working dog. Another example was where the two sons of a dog owner said they would not walk the dog down the street if it appeared it was castrated. Testosterone was for many years considered the reason for assertiveness in dog behaviour and this was then associated with a tendency to engage in fighting other dogs. All dog owners are familiar with the desire by male dogs to first sniff and then stop to squirt their urine onto any available vertical object. It was thought that this male behaviour would be reduced if a dog was castrated, but the behaviour of urine marking is imprinted and unless the puppy is neutered when it is quite young the urine making will still occur but less often than in the entire male.

Scent-marking hormones

Pheromones or 'scent hormones' are released in the urine, and there has been considerable research into trying to identify which chemical compounds in the urine are of the most importance in conveying messages. Urine-marking is seen even in neutered dogs, and it has also been observed that dogs will defecate in the centre of a path when in an unfamiliar locality. Such marking actions suggest that the behaviour is to provide a 'signpost' for a return route using scent marking, even where there were no vertical objects to mark. A further observation was made by another researcher that dogs tended to deposit solid faeces in a north-south direction, suggesting an inner body compass may be active.

Territorial scent and 'bioboundaries' are important to free-living canines in avoiding conflict between packs of dogs hunting for food. Signalling chemicals help a dog to recognise a location and also inform them about other dogs that have travelled the same way. This is of particular importance when dogs are exercised in parks and farmland which is frequented by other dogs. Hostile responses are sometimes inevitable when male dogs impinge on territory they consider to be their own. In a study of 100 guide dogs involved in random attacks recorded between 2006 and 2009, 97% of the attacks occurred in public areas. It was reported by Brooks in 2010 that in nearly half of the incidents the two dogs had first responded to each other in a friendly manner before the attack occurred. A high proportion of the guide dogs observed were displaying the appropriate dog-to-dog greeting behaviour before the attack occurred.

Pheromones secreted can induce unprovoked attacks. 60% of the attacked dogs were males, but as all guide dogs are neutered before one year old it should have reduced any testosterone aggression response. The colour and the breed of dog did not seem to be a reason why these guide dogs were attacked. The Labradors used were black and yellow, but fewer cross-bred Golden Retriever x Labradors were attacked than would have been anticipated statistically. It had previously been reported that other breeds with predominantly white coats were more subject to unprovoked attacks, something that is replicated in many species; in remote parts of Africa even albino children have been put to death in accordance with some primitive cultural tradition.

Fortunately assistance dogs trained for wheelchair users seem less likely to be attacked by other dogs, possibly because the person who does not have a visual disability is more able to avoid encounters with aggressive dogs.

The bull breed group formed 38% of the aggressor dogs in the attacked guide dog reports, but these encounters can be avoided or evasive action taken to avoid any direct approaches when threats are seen. Most of the aggressors were between one and six years old, when the highest hormone levels would be expected. It was not reported that any of the attacking dogs had been neutered.

Dominance is associated with testosterone secretion, and other hormones are involved such as adrenaline. The aggression facilitating effect of arginine vasopressin (AVP) appears to depend on testosterone and testosterone metabolites such as oestradiol and dihydrotestosterone. The testes just before and after birth produce a surge of testosterone that influences the subsequent development of the basic plan of mammals based on female characteristics. Again at puberty the male dog has a further surge of testosterone and male behaviour patterns develop.

Increased scent marking behaviour, inter-male aggression and secondary male characteristics are more obvious after this stage of development. About this age, dominance and later aggression may develop unless the dog is trained sensibly. When veterinary treatment was requested, resorting to medication with one of a number of antidepressant drugs was largely unsuccessful in treating owner-directed aggression. Neutering assistance dogs at an early stage in their training improves the dog's emotional tone and makes the task easier for reward based training methods.

Stress has been a subject much talked about, but it is not fully understood how the animal reacts to stressful situation such as those encountered on an almost daily basis by the working dog. Stress too will affect human health, as it influences the immune system and immunoglobulin levels in the blood. Women are more affected by chronic stress than men. Researchers at the University of Cincinnati found differing levels of stress hormone generated to aid survival and recovery are produced by the two sexes. The usual stress indicators are pulse, blood pressure and breathing rate. Taking samples of saliva from the mouth can be used to measure cortisol, a less invasive method than blood sampling. Salivary immunoglobulin A will alter within 20 minutes of stress exposure and can be used experimentally to see how people may be less stressed when a dog is present. Stress levels in the dogs being trained for assistance dog work have been measured using mouth swabs to measure cortisol in a limited study at the Banbury centre.

The support that can be given in difficult situations when an animal is present has been researched widely. One of the earliest 1997 studies in forensic psychology by Barker, was made on sexually-abused children; it was found that the subjects found animals more supportive than humans. The value of animal companionship for a child in a difficult situation cannot be underestimated; talking to a pet, touching and stroking the fur provide comfort from a non-judgmental subject, support something a human cannot easily provide or may not be so constantly present. Assistance animals with such children have been developed with Animal Assisted Activities (AAA), where a range of support is possible without necessarily involving 'interventions'. A child going into a clinic or hospital will have a reduced anxiety level when the assistance animal is permitted to be present. The physician can make a more detailed examination when the patient is not stressed and can understand the normal state of the patient who is less tense or frightened. In the following chapter you can read more about the support given to children (and adults) through the presence of a dog.

Chapter 11

Service dogs in many roles

'Service dogs' had been the term originally used in the United States for dogs trained to help in various sorts of disabilities. 'Service animals' were defined as dogs that are individually trained to work or perform tasks for people with disabilities (2011, US Department of Justice Disability Rights Section document). Such dogs were used after the Vietnam war in 1967, and in 2009 it was proposed to the US Senate that a 'Wounded Warrior K9 Corps' be set up with state funding for five years to provide dogs for veterans. It seemed like a new initiative giving official recognition to the help dogs could give, but now is the time to review the use of dogs to assist mankind in a historical context.

Long before those servicemen and women were given the possibility of having a specifically trained assistance dog, dogs had given assistance, right back to prehistory. In the earliest days of the hunter-gatherers, dogs were helping to pursue and drive game animals to be trapped or killed by hand-thrown weapons as shown on cave wall paintings. Dogs were also scavenging waste and providing an alerting bark or growl to warn persons of the approach of others, and all were part of the symbiosis developing between people and dogs.

Pictorial records of dogs assisting are non-existent, although fossil animal bones crunched by the powerful jaws of hyenas suggest that dogs too would obtain carcase food to live off.

Looking to the early religious records, Saint Jerome is credited with translating the Old Testament Bible from Hebrew into Latin. He was born in about 340 in Croatia whilst living a hermit-like existence for performing the translation; paintings often show him with a lion at his feet. The story recounted was that the two came to support each other after Jerome had removed a thorn from the animal's paw. Jerome was also known as a 'therapist', credited with treating a 20-year-old woman for possible anorexia. When he was chaplain to the aristocratic Blaesilla, he encouraged her to fast to death and then wrote to her mother saying she had been a victor in the struggle against Satan.

The stories seem hardly credible, but if one views the medieval artists' works, the 'lion' often has a dog-like face, suggesting that either the painters were not familiar with lions or they were implying it was a dog that was present during much of Jerome's years spent in the translation of this great work. It is suggested there had been a mistranslation of the animal. The Hebrew word 'keren', meaning rays of light, was misread as 'horns' in Exodus 34 when Moses came down from Mount Sinai, leading to medieval artists depicting Moses with horns! Perhaps in mis-translation, Jerome's assistance dog became a lion?

Even earlier than this there were accounts of the Greeks who kept dogs in their temples for healing, the writings advocating animal contacts such as horse riding for depression, known then as 'melancholy'. Dogs often appear in works of art; there are depictions of beggars seeking alms using dogs and possibly the dogs were mobility aids to blind people, as depicted by the engraver Dürer (1471–1528). Other paintings or accounts of dogs working with disabled persons have not been found, but dogs were trained in hunting and for guarding and defence.

In 1796, the Quakers set up an institution for mental disorders in York, as they were concerned at the inhumane treatment given to the insane or mentally disturbed. Dogs were present in the house as part of the more enlightened treatment; Sigmund Freud in Vienna often kept his dog in the consulting room when receiving patients, and dogs as 'assistants' in psychotherapy have often been used since.

Military service dogs

More recently there are records of the use of dogs assisting the vulnerable. In 1884 the German Army established a school training 'Sanitätshunde' (health dogs) to find wounded soldiers in the battlefields. When the First World War started in 1914, this army was already using dogs for rescue, sentry and messenger carrying. France had some 250 dogs enrolled for sentry and related duties and amongst the Allies; the Belgian army was using dogs to pull both Maxim guns and other supplies on wheeled carriages.

In the British sectors, 'service dogs' were introduced first to the trenches as companions and for alerting those sentries in the front lines, but they were not extensively used in assisting the military in their familiar work. I am indebted to Bruce Jones for information from his research into dogs used by the allies as well as the Germanic armies:

'Remarkably the War Office History of the veterinary services in the war, an impressive 800-page volume, only mentions dogs briefly in regard to repatriation in 1919. There is no official record of any veterinary services, possibly because in 1914 dogs had no recognised role, other than as regimental mascots. One report suggests that by 1918 Germany employed 30,000 dogs and Britain, France and Belgium over 20,000 (almost certainly a low figure) and Italy 3,000. Initially America did not use dogs, but took several hundred from the Allies for specific duties. Another source states that a million dogs were killed in action, but it is not qualified and appears high. Dogs were employed because of their intelligence, trainability and unique senses of smell and hearing, and in the trenches by soldiers for their companionship and loyalty.'

Rescue and Casualty Dogs, also called 'ambulance' or 'mercy' dogs were used by all armies. Red Cross dogs were trained to find casualties, then either to stay with the wounded man and bark, or to return to the handler to guide the ambulance team. Major Edwin Richardson established a War Dog Training School in Essex after the outbreak of war in 1914 and he preferred working with Airedales and Bloodhounds.

The scenting ability of dogs was used when poison gas warfare developed in 1915, as dogs could be trained to detect gas attacks before the soldiers were aware of the gas drifting on the wind and giving a warning to put on gas masks. There were even gas masks for dogs, as well as for the cavalry horses. In both world wars, dogs were either adopted or otherwise acquired as unit mascots and some played a valuable role in reducing the number of rats in the trenches of the Western Front of 1914-18. Dogs could provide mental diversions and companionship, as well as being a talisman against artillery shelling, and they could help focus troops on a task ahead as well as acting as effective guards against surprise attack.

In the 1939-1945 war, dogs were adopted by soldiers in prisoner of war camps and fed from the rations. Judy was such a dog, adopted by British prisoners held in one Japanese prison camp; she accompanied the POWs to their work places. Her warning growl alerted prisoners of the silent approach of guards, and she was a saviour for many suffering duress; the quoted remark as malnourishment sapped the energy of the unfortunate captives was 'If that bitch can do it, so can I'. The PDSA had identified the value of dogs in helping morale in war zones with the award of medals since 1943, and by 1947 there were 3000 such animals recognised.

Service dogs in the USA started in California as a response to the Americans with Disabilities Act in 1975. Once again, a war in a distant country lead to many amputees and disabled ex-servicemen, and many were found to obtain great benefit from being placed with a dog. The name 'service dog' in the USA had become prominent when used to assist injured soldiers and marines in Vietnam who had been able to have a dog trained for them. The name was not used in England, as it caused confusion with the army guard dogs trained by the British military as part of the armed services. The descriptive phrase 'assistance dog' became accepted terminology for this type of dog in Britain. The Americans with Disabilities Act included access rights for the 'service dogs', as their value had been proved beyond doubt.

Using ex-servicemen to train dogs was a further development in therapy. In February 2009, injured US soldiers at the Walter Reed Army Medical Hospital started training dogs under a 'Paws for Purple Hearts' (PPH) programme, and similar developments using disabled soldiers in England in the training of assistance dogs were being explored.

The geneticist Dr Joan Esnayra, President of the US Psychiatric Service Dog Society, said the bond between humans and canines went back to the Stone Age, and contact with dogs can release pleasure hormones in the brain. Trained dogs can also detect panic attacks and prevent them by calming the owner by close contact nuzzling or licking the person, producing a sense of stability and calm.

The Veterans Association in the USA had already undertaken an evaluation of the use of service dogs for individuals diagnosed with PTSD following the conflicts in Iraq and Afghanistan in 2011, and there were positive results. In England 'Veterans With Dogs' was set up as a charity in March 2013 specifically to train ex-service personnel who suffered from psychological injuries and PTSD to use assistance dogs trained for their needs. The charity also helps veterans to train their own dogs. Founded following the Afghanistan involvement, the charity also ran workshops seminars and residential activities in Devon. The charity is open to any person of any age who has served in the armed forces and currently has six dogs at work. Evidence-based research to gain a better base of symptoms and treatment goals besides conventional therapy is one of the objectives, they have worked with Dr Tracy Stecker, a psychologist at Dartmouth Medical School in the USA, a researcher into cognitive behavioural interventions in mental health situations; she has researched why dogs may help individuals with PTSD.

Hounds for Heroes was another new charity focused on dogs being specifically trained to assist injured service persons. The name was chosen for the training of dogs specifically for amputees and those with other injuries in uniformed service personnel; they also include those from emergency services such as the police who need assistance dogs. Alan Parton, as founder, had his own first assistance dog Endal trained by Canine Partners; he earlier acquired fame through his 'wonder dog', which at that time received extensive publicity through being able to operate an ATM cash machine.

In an address to the British Veterinary Association in Manchester in September 2014, Alan stated that he had trained 17 dogs to assist service people. He said he had started the organisation after having talked to a group of service people and set off to raise £20,000 as the cost of a dog throughout its life. He said the insurance for his own dog was costing him £80 a month, but the new charity would fully fund the dogs they trained for such expenses.

The rehabilitation centre at Headley Court is run by the Ministry of Defence for service personnel, and Alan had visited it to meet potential users of dogs; the charity was to be run by servicemen for their injured and disabled colleagues. In his talk, he said that once a building in Hampshire had been offered to him, he had started with the first six 'cadets', as the puppies were known; all had military-related names.

Later in his talk he spoke of placing some dogs with 'mad people', by which he meant the Post Traumatic Stress Disorder (PTSD) clients. They would also be included as one of the conditions of service people with which dogs would be trained to help. 'Reservist dogs' were also being used, not only for focusing on those injured today but because meeting the needs of all the potential clients was the priority.

A report in *The Times* two months later stated: 'an explosion of charities offering different and sometimes unproved treatment of veterans with mental illness could be harming rather than helping'. The commentary implied that there was a lack of regulation in treating PTSD in veterans. The same report stated that there were now more than 2000 military charities, including 370 that deal with mental health issues; collectively they were worth £1 billion.

Canine Partners for Independence was already having an active involvement with Headley Court, training a number of dogs for war veterans, and they were in receipt of funds from the larger charity Help for Heroes to pay to train specific dogs for servicemen. Dogs for the Disabled had earlier trained one dog with a very active disabled veteran and have a Trustee, Andy Lea from the Metropolitan Police service, who had suffered a severe neck injury. One proposal was for Dogs for the Disabled to investigate the possibility of dogs being used or be trained by PTSD service persons in conjunction with an Oxford-based researcher.

Puppies Behind Bars (PBB) was a prison guide dog programme started by veterinarian Dr Thomas Lane in America. Involving dogs in the rehabilitation of civilian prisoners had also been successful in Australia, based on similar projects in the USA. In Australia the Prison Pup Programme had about 35–40 dogs being trained in open prisons when Richard Lord spoke about the subject some years ago: it was 'open door work', not in cells but using small dormitories so the puppies got plenty of freedom.

'Puppies Behind Bars' described how a younger USA ex-serviceman was diagnosed with PTSD after three tours on the front line in Iraq. Mr Shaffer, aged 25, became a virtual recluse until he was given Megan, a Labrador from the USA programme. The same organisation that used convicted prisoners to train dogs for those with special needs over three years had placed dogs with soldiers with PTSD. Dogs were reported to help to curb paralysing activity such as panic attacks, and they also helped to get veterans back to work and reduce or abolish alcoholism. When the soldier experienced a return to drinking, then the next morning the dog could fetch medicine bottles with antidepressant or tranquillisers as a reminder to the patient of psychiatric support measures.

The idea of prisoners training dogs in England has also been explored in the West Midlands by Dogs for the Disabled, but when there was a change of the prison governor, difficulties were encountered in trying to develop dog training within the UK prison system. The USA charity idea that operates in 54 USA correctional facility prisons, was to be tried in a privately-run U K prison. The prisoners keep the dogs in their cells on week nights and the dogs spend weekends with handlers (often prison warders' families) in the outside world during their 12 to 18 months training. Unfortunately all the preliminary work was wasted after a change in the prison procedures.

Dog Aid

Other assistance dog charities were active in Britain but operating with less publicity. With a continuing demand for skilled companions, there were other ways of providing assistance dogs without involving the need for extensive funding for premises. Dog AID (Assistance Dogs in Disability) was a charity established in 1992 by Dolores Palmer and

John Rogerson to provide 'assistance in disability' by encouraging clients to train their own dogs. Their mission is to 'help those with physical disabilities which impair their movement and their ability to perform tasks such as picking up dropped objects, opening and shutting doors, finding articles that have been mislaid, putting washing in the machine, taking it out, placing articles where required, fetching help and many other tasks', to quote from their website.

New clients of Dog AID were required to find a young and trainable dog on their own. The head office in Shrewsbury would arrange to find a local approved trainer who would come to supervise and assist the dog to perform the required tasks. Local dog clubs would also be involved in support and attending classes was encouraged. The trainers were all volunteers who would bring the dog on to help the client reach assistance dog standard to meet the requirements of AD UK and be given access rights to a registered assistance dog. The scheme was practical and low cost, but required the continued involvement of the disabled owner in keeping up the training routine. Applicants had to be over 15 years old.

There was less waiting time than going to the larger established charities for assistance dogs; some owners chose to train for a replacement dog with higher ability next time, by getting their name on to the waiting list of one of the three more specialised assistant dog training charities.

Support Dogs

Support Dogs was founded in January 1992 by three ladies already involved in dog training, Linda Hams, Dolores Palmer and Val Strong. The charity was based on an idea of John Rogerson, a dog expert and author, as a result of his visit to the USA to observe assistance dogs in 'Top Dog', where owners had trained their own pets. He and his wife were the first Trustees; they helped disabled people with their own dogs. At first training was based on three areas around where the trainers lived, Sheffield, Staffordshire and Northamptonshire, where the first dogs were trained. The scheme started well, but then Linda Hams left to join Dogs for the Disabled at Tollgate House. Dolores Palmer went on to develop Dog AID through the country.

Support Dogs continued with Val Strong, and her first class of dogs were qualified in August 1993; training took place at various sites in Sheffield until permanent premises were obtained in 1997. Pedigree Petfoods sponsored the new organisation with £1500 for three years with publicity and leaflets. The Yorkshire-born personality Angela Rippon became the President in the first year of Support Dogs, and she opened Jessops Riverside Centre in 2005.

Claire Guest, then still with Hearing Dogs and later forming her own medical alert dogs' charity, was able to give advice to Support Dogs and many epilepsy detection dogs were successfully trained by Val Strong in Sheffield.

Disability Assistance Dogs were regularly trained, but the demand was sometimes greater than the training facility could deal with and like other charities in a similar position, it had to refuse more entries until funding improved. Support Dogs had moved to larger premises suitable to train more dogs in Jessops Riverside in 2005, but two years later the whole ground floor suffered from catastrophic flooding that affected large parts of Sheffield when the rivers burst their banks. Help came from many sources, and after a year it was possible to again resume training, so it was fully functional again when I visited the Chief Executive in 2010.

Support Dogs had successfully trained an autism assistance dog in 2008 and now continues to provide more dogs as one of only two charities specifically training for ASD children clients.

Seizure alert dogs can be trained to detect epilepsy and can effectively give up to 50 minutes' warning before an attack; years later came the first guide dog that detected epilepsy as a dual-purpose dog. Rita Howson, Support Dogs' Director of Operations said: 'We know Hetty is the first dog to deal with these two disabilities in the country, but we can find no mention of a similar dog anywhere else so we think she is totally unique and could be the first in the world. It is a remarkable testament to the growing relationship between Support Dogs and Guide Dogs'.

Hetty had been trained by the Guide Dogs for the Blind Association for Toni when she was two years old, and she was next trained by Support Dogs in Sheffield to detect an oncoming epileptic seizure in a blind person. Toni, 42, said: 'Hetty is a phenomenal dog, I could never have imagined how good she could be. Not only does she help guide me but she is always on the watch out for signs of a seizure. If it is a minor seizure she will come to a halt and sit, but at an offset angle, not straight like she normally does. If it is a major event, she will warn me by putting her chin on my knee or pawing at me. This gives me time to get to a place of safety'.

The Chief Executive of Guide Dogs, Richard Leaman, said: 'Dual dogs like Hetty transform the lives of people living with sight loss and other disabilities. This is a great example of two charities working together. We are confident that Hetty will help Toni live independently for many years to come and we look forward to doing more work with Support Dogs.'

By 2015, the GDBA had appointed an Additional Needs Manager who looks after the requirement by some blind people to have dual purpose dogs. The first such dog prepared was in 2003 for Angela, who had severe hearing loss as well as loss of vision.

Pauline Williams had been trained with a black Labrador, Susannah, in March 1991. Previously a guide dog owner, she could not get a replacement after her diabetes developed complications. I visited her in her home in Cardiff in May 1995, as she had the unique combination of having both legs amputated below the knees and she had lost three fingers as well as being blind. She lived in sheltered accommodation, using her wheelchair with Susannah besides her; she could travel along a paved veranda to call on friends when she wanted company. She lived close to Ely Hospital and her Labrador was trained by Dogs for the Disabled after the dog had been obtained from the Forfar GDBA centre as one suited for a less active role.

Medical Detection Dogs

This innovative and successful charity was started by Claire Guest, a graduate in Psychology trained at Swansea University. She had joined Hearing Dogs for the Deaf in its early days when they were based at Aston Rowant near the Chiltern Hills under the directorship of Tony Blunt. Claire, starting in the early 1990s, progressed with this form of assistance dog training and I watched her demonstrate her skill in 2001 at the kennels at Cliffe in Yorkshire. She had been successful in training hearing dogs for a number of years and she already wanted to train a dog for an epileptic patient, which she did in her own time whilst living near Aylesbury.

Hearing Dogs for Deaf Persons had by then moved from the Lewknor Kennels to a much larger purpose-built facility. The Grange, as the new Chiltern base, opened in 2002. Organisational changes at HDFD, which after thirty years had gained recognition and financial stability, led Claire to look into the possibility of becoming involved in a new organisation that would find out how dogs' olfactory senses could provide help in some human diseases.

Whilst still working as a trainer/instructor for this large charity, Claire started preparing a dog in her own time to seek out disease in humans. This was a new application for assistance dogs based on the very fine scent discrimination of a dog. As might be expected, the gundog breeds, which had had many generations of selection for finding game birds and shot animals, were the most proficient when various breeds were considered. Dogs were also trained to detect epileptic fits, so this was one of the two organisations, the other being Support Dogs, that did this type of detection. Claire trained dogs to detect prostate cancer signs in urine samples.

Her work with Dr Church and colleagues was published. An earlier report had been of a Dalmatian in 1987 which had detected a malignant melanoma, a workplace anecdote which he wrote about in the medical journal *The Lancet* in 1989. The report brought a lot of interest in the possibility of using dogs to detect other conditions. Dr Church said in 2001, 'Fortunately a scientific approach was used and dogs' success rates were recorded'. This allowed for further publications in prestigious magazines read by medical workers in England and elsewhere in the world.

A report on dogs scenting compounds in urine specimens to predict bladder cancer was published in the *British Medical Journal* in 2004, stating a 91% success rate in the trained dogs compared with as low as 14% if only random detections were taking place. Medical Detection Dogs became a registered charity in 2008, after Claire and her supporters had raised sufficient funds to convince the charity commissioners that this was a charity with a future. There are two arms to the charity: the cancer detection arm and the medical assistance dog arm. Once trained, the diabetes type detection dogs were registered as assistance dogs, which gave them the same access rights to transport and food stores etc enjoyed by guide dogs and now several other groups. This was especially necessary for all the different medical alert dogs Claire was training. 'Diabetes hypo alert dogs' were the most frequently called for, as they were found to be of great help to those diabetics who had fluctuating levels of sugar in their blood; insulin injections were not working with frequent changes in the dose and frequency of injections. If the insulin worked too well, then the glucose level fell and the diabetic person might collapse with hardly any warning. The trained dogs could detect odours and even small changes in behaviour in the person and alert them in time to take food that would restore the blood sugar level. Similarly when blood sugar levels rose above normal (hyperglycaemia), the dog could alert the owner in various ways by barking, licking or jumping up. The dog could next fetch any medical supplies, often carried by the owner in a rucksack or wallet. Furthermore, the fact that the dog wore a jacket, showing it was a trained alert dog, meant that any member of the public coming across a prone or unconscious person with the dog close too would know to call for medical help rather than passing by 'just another drunk on the floor'.

Besides their use in diabetes detection, dogs' discriminating sense of smell can be applied to detecting changes in patients suffering with Addison's disease. The condition is life-threatening, with sudden collapse, which means that patients may have to be admitted into hospital. Collapse can occur in a crisis situation, and severe pain and convulsions may follow, with unconsciousness as the blood pressure drops down. In this life-threatening situation, a dog can bring the vital medical treatment and its presence allows paramedics to be called for quickly.

A further use for a medical alert dog was to help a 17-year-old with narcolepsy, involving a sudden sleep sensation and paralysis, a condition that makes it difficult to leave the home without a human escort. The client was being prepared to have a trained dog 'on call' 24 hours a day, allowing a release from a sense of imprisonment, with all the other benefits of greater activity. Training similar dogs could cause savings in the National Health service: in 2012-13, there were 345 hospital admissions of patients with narcolepsy whilst others were treated at home. There are 55 medical alert assistance dogs out with clients in 2014, trained by Claire's charity and nearly 40 more coming through their puppy socialising and training schemes.

Another success was four-year-old Rebecca, a brittle diabetic who had the first dog to enter a primary school officially in Northampton. Twelve dogs have now been trained, Claire told me when I visited her, and there have been more since then. Rebecca, with Shirley, her 'hypo-alert' dog, was featured in the national press in 2010.

Bio-Medical Detection Dogs is the name registered for disease biodetection (such as cancer). Research into the potential use of dogs to 'assist medics in the early detection and diagnosis of human disease' was undertaken by Claire Guest. Using urine samples in prostate cancer detection, one dog was found to be very good at it early on, and there was also accuracy in melanoma detection. Over two and a half years, six dogs trained for the detection of prostate cancer achieved a high success rate: 90% accuracy was possible, it was found during urological dog testing. Training was based on the positive reward system: as soon as the young dog indicates the correct urine specimen from a cancer patient, an audible click is followed by a small food reward, or later perhaps just vocal praise.

The dog's nose

Testing relies on the dog's unique ability to discriminate odours. The breeds selected over many generations to work and hunt have the best-developed scenting abilities. Volatile organic compounds (VOCs) in urine have been proposed as cancer biomarkers. The published description of one project to evaluate the efficacy of prostate cancer was based on detection by trained dogs on human urine samples. A Belgian Malinois Shepherd was trained by the clicker training method (operant conditioning) to scent and recognize the urine of people having prostate cancer. There was no testing of the people, but their urine samples were frozen for preservation and heated to the same temperature for all tests.

After the dog's learning phase and the training period of the two-year-old, the dog's ability to discriminate between prostate cancer and control urine was tested. Using a double blind procedure, urine was obtained from 66 patients referred to a urologist for elevated prostate-specific antigen (PSA) or abnormal digital rectal examination. All patients underwent prostate biopsy for diagnosis and two groups were considered: 33 patients with cancer and 33 controls presenting negative biopsies. Urine samples were presented to the dog to sniff on a rotary device to carry a number of specimens for the dog to test. During each 'run' the dog was asked to signal a cancer urine among six samples containing only one cancer urine and five randomly-selected controls. In this report the dog completed all the runs and correctly indicated the cancer samples in 30 of 33 cases. Of the three cases wrongly classified as cancer, one patient was rebiopsied and prostate cancer was confirmed.

The detection of specific volatile organic compounds could be used as screening method for early detection of prostate cancer. Dogs' scenting ability was tested by using dilutions of a chemical, amyl acetate, which has a strong odour: at a dilution of 1 part in a trillion a trained dog was still able to recognise the correct sample.

Research into detecting volatile particles associated with breast cancer using dogs' scent discrimination will require a large number of specimens to test the breath of 216 patients. There are many other possibilities for applying the dogs' scenting abilities, such as the three dogs trained to sniff out bedbugs in hostels and at other sleeping facilities. Canine interactions can be used in assistance dog work far beyond the idea of Frances Hay and other pioneers.

Community dogs

Various organisations train dogs for specialised tasks, often relying on scenting ability, but although a form of service dog, they are outside the scope of this book. Community Dogs is a new activity set up by Dogs for the Disabled where the full-time ownership of a dog is not practicable. The Kingswood Trust supervises residential facilities for adults with autism. A dog and an instructor have been present since 2010, first as a weekly visit, but now attends full time; the instructor previously worked for Hearing Dogs for Deaf People. At the Trust's one location, they are assisting with four adults, and the work was appreciated by Kingswood, who fund most of the costs. The dogs can teach road safety, and have a calming influence, encouraging a more stable lifestyle. Those with limited verbal communication skills found that talking to the dog encouraged them to communicate where the dog did not expect a high standard of speech. A certificate in animal care was introduced, with a course that gives adults the chance to learn for a specific goal.

In the spring of 2014, Dogs for the Disabled began a new community scheme at two special educational needs schools in the Midlands. An instructor attends with her community assistance dog to help with the children. The presence of a dog interests the children and has an 'impact on personal and social skills' and 'will have a positive impact across the school'. A second school further away in Buckinghamshire is also using a community dog. The Child Brain Injury Trust, based at Bicester near to the Frances Hay Centre, has also found the benefits of a community dog to understand the importance of road safety. Parents of children with acquired brain injury supported the idea of a helping dog and one pilot scheme was set up with a seven-year-old boy who received a visit once a week for eight weeks by Lana with the instructor, to see how Animal Assisted Activities (AAA) might be of benefit. Further developments with other children are possible.

Dementia Dogs developed as a pilot exercise in Scotland. It started as a Glasgow School of Art service design project commissioned by Alzheimer Scotland: Action on Dementia. Assistance dog charities were approached and the GDBA and Dogs for the Disabled took on the new challenge, since both were interested in this form of disability. Four dogs were assessed for suitability and were trained at the Forfar GDBA centre. Four families where one partner was affected and suitable to receive one of the trained Dementia Dogs were found locally. They received regular visits from Dogs for the Disabled's trainers and from the Alzheimer's Society local staff. Starting in June 2013, there were three units functioning 18 months later and their progress was carefully monitored. The experiences will be assessed after two years and a decision taken on whether to expand the use of this type of assistance dog as further funding became available in 2015.

Chapter 12

Children with special needs and assistance dogs

Assistance Animal Interventions (AAI) is the term currently used where selected dogs are helping children and others with special needs. Although dogs have always been used in this way in families as companions for children, it is only when specially chosen and often individually trained dogs are used that the maximum benefit with AAI for the child can be obtained.

The range of disorders, both physical and mental, where dogs can help is extensive. The next chapter will deal specifically with autism spectrum disorders, but many other situations where dogs have helped children can be considered here. Some years ago in 1971, the role of a canine therapist in a residential children's setting, where it was known as 'pet facilitated therapy' in the USA, was described by Loney. The first child to be trained by Bonita Bergin in the USA with an assistance dog was for a six-year-old boy, Kristofer Ledwick, in 1983. He was said to have a dog that responded to 88 words of command, but there was some disbelief amongst dog trainers in England that this was possible for a dog.

In the *National Geographic World* magazine in August 1985, there was an account of a boy who had learned to give his service dog, Ivy, 88 commands. When this was brought to the attention of trainers who were used to a very few commands such as 'sit' and 'stay' in the UK, scepticism followed. It was pointed out that more word responses could be obtained by linking word sounds together, which allowed the dog to distinguish 219 objects and actions. 'Fetch blue' would make the dog go to a pile of objects and bring back the correct colour object without distinguishing the command. Whilst Dogs for the Disabled never claimed this large vocabulary recognition for the dogs trained in the 1990s, Canine Partners were able to say the dogs they trained could be as good as the 1985 American dog in responding to many such words.

Dogs for the Disabled's first training with children began in 1989. In the early days of the charity, one of Frances' more ambitious projects was to train a Standard Poodle as an assistance dog for a tiny child with severe disabilities. Mary Ann was the size of a three year old with matchstick arms and legs but a well-developed head, larger in proportion than the rest of her body. She was alert and intelligent and had devoted parents, who came up from North London to Kenilworth for the residential training of the poodle Max with their daughter. Frances had obtained the free loan of a bungalow and garden in Kenilworth, so the family could live close at hand whilst Max was brought in to them each day.

Max had been specifically purchased and delivered to puppy socialisers on March 5th 1989 to prepare him for assistance dog training. He was almost fully grown and had a tight black curly coat, and it was thought that there would be no risk to the child from boisterousness nor from allergy to the dog's close-clipped coat. The parents were delighted with Mary Ann's interest in the dog; she could throw a small ball whilst sitting up in her chair, which the dog would retrieve and bring back each time to place it in her lap. She never seemed to tire of the game, and even when someone else threw the ball as she was watching the dog, it gave her far more variety than any mechanical game or when she was looking at the 'mobile' suspended above her, as had been previously tried.

The dog had been socialised at first to go out as a companion dog for an elderly person, but then was used by Frances for Mary Ann. After a fortnight Frances supervised Max's handover, having personally visited the family in the bungalow every day. I visited Max to 'qualify' him before the family and child returned with Max as assistance dog to their London home. I had been to meet the parents twice during their stay in Kenilworth and on qualifying the dog discussed health and veterinary care for Max. He was listed as the 17th dog trained, but was retired after the first year when his young 'partner' passed on. The charity Trustees agreed the parents would be allowed to keep the dog rather than calling it back in for reissue, as they had such pleasant memories of Max spending time with their young daughter.

Marty, a Collie cross that Frances prepared for a 13-year-old girl with spina bifida, was another early success with matching a dog to a child with special needs. There was no possibility of using the loaned bungalow again. A new location was provided by the Helen Ley Charity, between Kenilworth and Leamington, a purpose-built and well-equipped respite home for multiple sclerosis patients. The manager was willing to accommodate Abigail and the dog Marty, as there were suitable hoists and special equipment that helped disabled people to get around. The training was successful, with Caroline coming as the trainer each day from Coventry to work with Marty, and having a dog about the respite home was popular with the older people staying there for respite care.

When Abigail returned to Cheshire after just over two weeks at Helen Lay House, Abigail's mother was pleased with the greater independence shown by her daughter with Marty there as her constant attendant. The dog was qualified in Cheshire in December 1989 and Frances would have known how successful this team of child and dog had become. Sadly Frances was not there to see how well the dog developed in the years ahead for Abigail as her assistance dog, which later enabled her to get to study at college.

At about this time there was another anonymous tribute to Frances' work from the mother of a daughter with congenital muscular dystrophy, who had received a dog. 'All she wanted to do when she was in hospital was to see the dog, she was so ill that they let us take him in to the intensive care ward,' she said. 'The doctors took pictures and one has done lectures and shown the pictures to the students. My daughter really adores the dog – he is her whole life – and I think it is due to him that she has recovered.'

Frances Hay had a natural affinity for working with children, and her own daughter Debora had been brought up with dogs around her in the home. When Frances started in Kenilworth in 1988, she had said on the radio she wanted to place a few trained dogs with younger people, and some parents applied through local contacts, while other requests from further afield came in. There were even more enquiries after Frances appeared in the popular TV show Blue Peter, which had a long connection with assistance dogs through Derek Freeman of the Guide Dogs for the Blind Association; he had become a personal friend of the producer Biddy Baxter.

In 1964, Derek had taken to the BBC London TV studios a Labrador puppy, Honey, which had already been chosen as a future guide dog. The two regularly appeared on the show from then onwards, giving children the opportunity to see a dog developing and then being trained as an assistance dog. Valerie Singleton and Christopher Trace were the presenters at that time and then for the second dog that replaced Honey, Peter Purves, fresh from appearing in Doctor Who, took charge of her on the show and years later he kept up a connection with Dogs for the Disabled. Later, he came to Kenilworth to start off a sponsored dog walk where a memorial bench was unveiled to the accompaniment of music from Cubbington Silver Band. Peter was appointed a Vice-Patron in October 2001.

It was through this connection that Frances was invited by the BBC to the London TV studios to demonstrate with Amanda and Poppy as another sort of assistance dog. Frances had the hope that publicity would help to bring more funds in as well as recognition of her work with children. Unfortunately, after Frances' death in 1990, only a few more children were trained with dogs and for many years the Trustees rather frowned on getting involved in AAI activities. The guide dog organisation then had a 'no clients under 18 years old' rule and the trainers were very much of the thinking that working assistance dogs were only for adults.

Social dog Zoe: an assistance dog for Naomi

This account of a dog placed with an eleven-year-old girl with cerebral palsy in the early years of Dogs for the Disabled was written by her mother:

'In January 1989 my children and I were watching one of our favourite programmes, Blue Peter, when there appeared an item on the charity Dogs for the Disabled featuring a pretty Labrador cross Border Collie called Poppy. We were a single-parent family at the time. My daughter Naomi was eleven and attended a special school at Bradford, and her brother James was a very lively seven years old. Naomi was a premature baby who was very slow to achieve her developmental 'milestones' (sitting up, crawling etc.) and was diagnosed with cerebral palsy at the age of 18 months. She has never learnt to walk unaided but mobilises around the house with tripod sticks, using a wheelchair out of doors.

'As well as her physical disabilities, Naomi has visual impairment and learning difficulties. However she is very articulate and sociable, and likes nothing better than socialising with friends and family. We were already thinking about having a dog to enrich our family life, so I wrote off to Frances Hay in Kenilworth using the address given. I then had to fill in an application form and after a short delay and a few phone calls I heard that I would be visited by Dick Lane early in September of that year. We were not looking for a specially-trained dog but one with a pleasant nature who would be a companion for Naomi and the family.

'We discussed with Mr Lane what we were looking for and after another two months we heard he would be bringing Zoe up to us. When she arrived one late afternoon she was a beautiful long-haired Collie Cross Whippet. She had been donated to DFD and received three weeks' intensive training before being placed with us. Zoe turned out to be a lovable, submissive dog and soon settled in as part of the family. She was gentle with Naomi and walked beautifully alongside the wheelchair on our walks, whatever the weather. Naomi enjoyed sitting quietly with Zoe and stroking her, and was happy to talk to people about her 'special' dog. James enjoyed the companionship of a dog in the family and would walk her in the countryside around our house, often with his friends. Zoe was much admired and petted!

'Zoe always accompanied us on our annual holidays to see my parents in Cornwall and it was there that we met another recipient of a trained dog from DFD, Shep, a border collie placed with Ann Greenwood who was also a wheelchair user. I remember being very impressed with Shep's talents - he could 'answer' the phone, help fill the washing machine and even assist Ann in tacking up her driving ponies! We had some lovely photos of the two dogs playing together in Ann's garden that afternoon; they made a very handsome couple.

'Then in 1991 we were involved in making a video on Assistance Animals – I remember the filming took place in our local park with a cameraman who had travelled up from the London veterinary college. Naomi was interviewed on camera and Zoe enjoyed the next part, where she had to retrieve the sticks thrown in the park from the wheelchair. We were later invited to the launch of the video at the Royal Veterinary College in Camden Town; David Blunkett with his black Labrador guide dog was the chief guest. He spoke about the value of the different sorts of assistance dogs after being first introduced by the film's director, Jenny Poland, who was also a vet.

'When Naomi went on to residential college in 1995, Zoe was semi-retired but remained a much-loved member of the family. We had been having a visit once a year up until then, sometimes by Dick or on occasions a Middlesbrough trainer who was more accustomed to seeing guide dogs at work!

'Sadly Zoe was diagnosed with cancer of the liver earlier in 1995 but received exceptional treatment from our local vet and was able to live happily for another two years. When it finally became necessary to put her to sleep there were many tears shed! We had some lovely memories of the fun and enjoyment.'

In many ways this had been the ideal match of a 'surplus or rescue dog' with a family looking for an assistance dog. When I first met Zoe she was in a room on the second floor of a block of council flats. I had a recollection of a very long lounge, just a few pieces of furniture and a baby on a settee, at the far end of the room. The single mother had been used to animals in her family home and after the baby was born she had been allocated this flat in a fairly bleak area in the suburbs by the City of Coventry housing department.

I soon found that Zoe was not only used to going for walks on a lead beside the pram, ideal as it turned out as preparation for a wheelchair user, but was very clean in the house. Zoe's owner had trained her well but had to get rid of the dog as it was in community housing with rules on pet ownership. Frances heard about a dog needing rehoming and once a suitable placement was found, it was arranged that Zoe would be collected and go to Frances Hay's own Kenilworth house for 21 days' training and acclimatisation. The day I went to collect Zoe, I found she had been moved out of the flat to her owners' parents living nearby. It was obvious she was equally at home living there with the larger extended family, so socialisation had been more than adequate to prepare for her next move.

In the earliest days in Kenilworth, Dogs for the Disabled were mainly using abandoned dogs, some from dogs' homes or rescue kennels. Others like Zoe were offered direct to the charity, which was much preferred as it provided information on where that dog might be most suited to go. Francis used a wheelchair when she trained Zoe in Kenilworth to go out for walks, and her helpers would sit quietly during the wheelchair training sessions. Zoe, already used to going out beside the pram, performed so well that soon I arranged to deliver her, on one of my regular visits north to Sheffield, where my son was at university. Zoe stayed at home with me overnight and was no trouble on the long car journey north beyond Sheffield, eventually arriving at Naomi's home near Bradford in the late afternoon. She quite accepted her new placement and after a few formalities was left in the care of her very nice new family.

Telephone contacts continued but it was quite obvious that Zoe had 'landed on her feet'. I saw her on several 'aftercare' visits in the years after her successful placement. When contacted by some people from a companion animals study group, the 'tasks' Zoe could perform did not meet up with the type of AAI activity that dogs in the USA were trained up to and the dog's role was rather dismissed. Fortunately Jenny Poland had a small budget for educational films and heard about Zoe and AAI. When enough money was obtained to make a promotional film on assistance dogs by the Royal Veterinary College's film unit, the choice of Naomi and Zoe was an obvious one. Bruce Fogle and Neil Ewart were consulted, amongst others, on making the film. The film would show different assistance dogs at work, and it could also show how the introduction of an assistance dog could have a positive effect in a family with a special needs child and the benefits that a loving companion dog like Zoe can bring into family life.

The film was launched at a reception at Camden Town College and the local MP with his guide dog was able to attend as one of the invited guests. He spoke about the value of dogs after the showing of the film and met three types of Dogs for the Disabled dogs - Ben with Gina Geary, Elton with Debby Parry and Zoe with Naomi Sills.

More assistance dogs with children: Bodie & Curtis

After the death of Frances, the Trustees in charge of Dogs for the Disabled at first continued with the policy of training both children and adults with dogs. In September 1991, Caroline Fraser interviewed a 12-year-old boy who lived with his single-parent mother and a younger brother. Affected by muscular dystrophy, Richard had continued attending school. He had only the use of his hands but he could control and use an electric wheelchair for mobility. There was a requirement to train a dog that could lift the boy's right arm onto the arm rest of the wheelchair where the control lever was.

Richard was described as bright and cheerful and quite confident with people, and his mother hoped that owning a dog would boost his self-esteem, which was 'beginning to flag'. Bodie, the Collie-type dog provided, worked well and was a confidence builder for the boy, but dogs were was not allowed to enter the school and this rule was enforced. At that time Duchenne muscular dystrophy usually resulted in death by the late teens, but the dog was considered to have been good for the boy in his home. The partnerships proved a success and led to further placements of dogs with young men who also had muscular dystrophy diagnosed.

Within the disability network, word was passing round that dogs were of benefit and more enquiries came in for dogs. Gareth, also with muscular dystrophy, had been using an electric wheelchair since the age of eight and after losing his own pet Labrador in 1991 he heard from a friend's magazine about the new assistance dog organisation. He applied, was interviewed by the trainer Angie and after several visits she brought Curtis, a two-year-old trained Labrador, to his home in North Wales. There was an immediate match, and he described his dog as 'charming, affectionate, very intelligent and a real character too'.

He had his own flat attached to his parents' house and Curtis was trained to bring the special environmental control system arm to him where he could reach it. On the command 'Pull possum', Curtis could use his head to nudge Gareth's hand to the control box if Gareth lost his grip. As Curtis settled down to the new home, the two worked together to discover new ways to help Gareth: by opening and closing the garden gate, pulling the door stops away from doors wedged open, turning on and off the special heat-sensitive light switch and bringing various items directly to Gareth.

After the showing of the film in London, a request came from the Welsh TV studios in Bangor for a discussion programme about assistance dogs. Some clips from the film were used and it was arranged for Gareth to appear live on the international TV transmission from Caernarvonshire in North Wales. The studios were within half an hour of Gareth's home and they had an interactive link with a school in Brittany.

Curtis impressed everyone with his confidence with Gareth in a new situation. The good behaviour of the dog beside Gareth under the bright lights facing several technicians moving the cameras was exceptional. We sat in a row of chairs facing the interviewer. Questions came in from the French schoolchildren: Gareth said one of the most important things to him having a dog was that he could express affection. He said his previous pet dog was always out of reach if he wanted to stroke him, but Curtis would jump up on the bed or get to his level in the wheelchair and he said there was 'nothing like one of Curtis's big cuddles'. The feeling of safety, he said, was also important, as Curtis would bark on command and find help if needed, either running next door to get one of the family or upstairs for a carer.

The independence the dog gave him was important; he could go into his kitchen on a dark winter's night, somewhere previously 'out of bounds', as without help there was no one to turn on the light. The relationship meant that the dog was dependent on Gareth to feed him, walk him out and look after him; in return he was always there ready, eager to please and help Gareth. The half-hour programme went well and we felt we had taken the first step towards promoting assistance dogs in Europe.

Gareth had a schoolfriend, Tony, living in South Wales, who had the same muscular disorder; he was able to obtain an assistance dog trained from the Exeter guide dog centre, as the word passed round of the help that could be given by a dog. Dogs for the Disabled had been offered a dog unsuited for guide dog work which was thought could be suited for a wheelchair user. Tony became the unfortunate owner of Arran, described in Chapter 5. The dog underwent a surgical procedure that evidently did not progress as expected and was put to sleep on the Monday following the hip operation the previous Friday. Tony was not informed of the dog's progress over the weekend and only found out his dog was dead by a phone call on the Monday evening, as was stated in the subsequent County Court case at Cardiff. Judge North ascertained the dog had been euthanased without consent, although it was said in the evidence that attempts had been made to phone Tony during that day.

Tony was extremely distressed at the loss of his dog and when he found out about the death, he phoned George Cram, the instructor at the Exeter centre. A home visit was made by George to Tony and priority was given to obtaining a replacement dog as quickly as possible. It was an incident that should never have happened, and I am glad to say I never saw or heard of such a situation again.

With elderly or infirm dogs the client owner is usually prepared for the dog's end and practical support is given as far as possible when the time comes. The question was often asked, what happens when the child becomes an adult and secondly, what is the effect of losing a dog through death or accident? Tony was just very unfortunate person and eventually he passed away himself, as a result of the Duchene muscular dystrophy.

A more recent and happier tale comes from Hollie, now in her early twenties, who was first trained with assistance dog Hilton when she was 16; at that age her mother had to be legally responsible as the 'carer'. Hollie trained at home with Hilton; the instructor, Louise, found Hollie was quick to learn what Hilton could do to help her fetch and carry. Hollie had no effective use of her arms, but she had a confident voice, so hand signals were not necessary when using reward training.

Two years later, still living at home in her mother's house, Hollie was retrained, with Hilton now taking the part of an adult in sole charge of her assistance dog. I already knew about the dog, as he was sponsored by the hotel group who had helped Dogs for the Disabled with substantial financial input. When I met the partnership in 2014, I asked Hollie how she came to apply for a dog as a young person. She said she had seen a teenager on the TV show Children in Need and realised that was exactly what she wanted. After making enquiries she went across to the Dogs for the Disabled centre at Nostell near Halifax and met many others working with their dogs. She had talked to Louise and found out what the dogs could do.

From the first enquiry it took just under two years before she received the very attractive Hilton, who I was glad to see she had kept slim and not overfed with treats. Hollie was hoping to achieve full independence, with her own accommodation where she could keep herself and her dog, as they were a successful working partnership.

Physical health improvement and dog ownership

The reports about the children who had received assistance dogs all indicated that there was an improvement in their health after receiving their dogs. There have now been a considerable number of research reports coming in from the USA and Europe that showed that assistance dogs were beneficial in many ways to children with disabilities. When I first went out to Warsaw in 2004 to meet animal trainer Maria, I was shown how her large Husky-sized dogs were regularly taken into schools for deaf children, and anecdotally they were seen to be having a good influence on the children's social skills.

I had been invited there to give a talk titled *Angielski prawodawstwo dotyczace psow* (English assistance dogs) to the delegates at the Polish CZE-Ne-Ka Conference, describing the dog work with children in England. It needed good interpreters with skill to translate as I spoke. Several of them have remained friends since my visits, especially Magadalena, who I found had the same disability as our founder, Frances Hay. In Warsaw children were sent to a 'special school for severely handicapped'. As one person described it at the conference, there were state institutions with scarcely any lessons, and music and craft were used to fill the day. Dogs provided an outlet for social stimulation. When keyboards became more available there were new opportunities for the special needs children. They could start communicating more, which allowed for more independence and a way of showing how their world was perceived. Pets too allowed freedom of expression. The child senses if it is going too far in a 'rough and tumble' session with a dog or cat and knows when to allow a cooling-off period in active play.

For a period of nearly ten years Dogs for the Disabled had trained no child partnerships, until a parent who had been to the USA persuaded the charity Trustees to train a dog for an 11-year-old boy, Tom, and he was qualified with Labrador Vigo in December 2004. Tom became one of the first children in the UK to become registered with an assistance dog. He was about to move into secondary school and his mother was the appointed official 'carer' in the partnership; she was an enthusiastic supporter of assistance dogs and it was even suggested she might be invited to join the Trustee board.

Another dog was trained with a young girl, Kayleigh, who I first met with her dog when both young people came to visit Crufts Show the following spring. During the press invitation event, both children kept their heads down, but they were able to look at their dogs rather than just keeping their eyes on the floor as has been seen previously. The presence of the dogs helped to overcome any shyness when coming for the first time to a large event.

The children's project then got the 'go-ahead', with more dog partnerships planned in 2005. There was an opportunity to observe changes in the children's physical capabilities; confidence, bolder speech, general mood and ability to play with the dog were also to be observed. Dr June McNicholas from the University of Warwick gave advice on the therapeutic benefits expected in these partnerships. Unfortunately, due to timing, the opportunity to research these improvements in the children was lost. It was to take many more years before a research project on sociability and other benefits for children could be set up and a source of finance for it found.

There were already published research reports from the Netherlands of work by Marie-Jose Enders-Siegers that proved that companion animals do have an influence on the emotional and cognitive development of children. The children were found to be more relaxed in the presence of a pet and pets provided social support. In the Netherlands, specially trained 'guide dog' types of dog were being used for autistic spectrum disorder children to 'enhance their quality of life' in one project involving 11 dogs. Enders-Siegers research in the Netherlands followed on the earlier successful projects in Canada and Ireland with autism; in both countries dogs unsuited to work for blind people as guides were retrained as dogs to help young children.

Marie-Jose Enders-Siegers had been observing several Labradors aged 1½ years placed with families that had an autistic child. All the families had an initial interview and then kept diaries for the six months, usually filled in by the mothers. A period of observation ended with a further interview with the family. It was interesting that she could report on any partnership 'failures' such as any new programme might encounter. One dog had to be immediately withdrawn as the child 'could not stand the smell' of the dog.

In the other 10 dogs placed with children aged between four and seven, three girls and nine boys, nine of the dogs were considered a success. One boy became very aggressive and the dog was withdrawn on welfare grounds, but the other combinations all showed positive results. The mobility of the children increased and social behaviour too improved with the children showing more interest in their environment and the parents reported development of speech and eye contact. There was increased relaxation in these Dutch families; one mother said 'we are a normal family again' and siblings were especially appreciative of the assistance dog that came to live in their home.

The research was demonstrating that not every dog placement would be a success, but overall the benefits were there for this type of assistance dog work. The close contact with the dog at the same eye level as the child, the child's hands easily touching the dog's hair and the dog acting as a social facilitator with other people were all considered factors in the improvements observed. Cultural differences and attitudes could be a problem; in Holland one mother did not like to be seen in public with her child and the assistance dog as this she felt labelled her unfairly, and this problem had been encountered in England as well. Yet even amongst people who do not own pets themselves, pets can act as a social lubricant or 'ice breaker'. A cared-for dog invited comment, giving a neutral topic to open a conversation with someone passing by in the street, whilst the same person would not stop to talk about the child for fear of being seen to be critical of the child's behaviour.

Noses and paws

Touching an animal is easy for a child, especially when the dog's size is close to that of the child. Such physical contacts are important developmentally, and research has shown that even newborn babies are incredibly sensitive to pleasurable touch. The inquisitive dog will often place its nose gently on a child, and sometimes face licking follows. Researchers at the Max Planck Institute for Cognitive and Brain Sciences in Germany recently showed that the bond between parent and infant could be enhanced by the infant's 'unique physiological and behavioural responses'.

Some people with autism are under-responsive to sensory stimuli as well as having a lack control of their actions. A head or nose contact with a child having an ASD 'tantrum' or a head-banging session, will often stop it. Petting a dog with gentle stroking or just touching the head in passing increases fine motor skills; the presence of the dog helps to improve sensory perception, relating to how the dog feels about the contact. The child can develop with the knowledge that the dog will be constantly present or waiting to greet them after an absence at school. Sometimes the first words a 'non-verbal' child speaks will be addressed to the dog, or will be about something the dog has done. Social interactions with others, language skills can all improve after a dog comes into the family.

Evidence from research worldwide confirms that there are beneficial effects for children interacting with dogs. The 2005 IAHAIO conference report stated that scientific evidence supports the beneficial effects of interactions with companion animals for human health and wellbeing. The quality of the evidence, however, was often questioned. Research became a priority in further work with British children and Dogs for the Disabled, with the help of Professor Daniel Mills at Lincoln University, were able to obtain a three-year research grant from the Big Lottery Fund. The work was done with the autism charity on children diagnosed with ASD and their families, comparing those who had a trained dog with other families where there was no dog in the home. In the research based at Lincoln University, working closely with Dogs for the Disabled and NAS (National Autistic Society), one striking and almost constant feature was that members of the family around the autistic child felt more relaxed and were less challenged by daily events once the dog was present in the home. The research results, published in 2015, showed statistically that in those families which took on a dog where there was a child with ASD, stress levels were consistently reduced. Strangely enough, the child in this situation will often refer to 'my dog' and when out for walks attached by a waistband to the assistance dog, the child gives the impression of being the one in charge, even though the parent has the much longer lead attached to the dog. Benefits in companionship are obvious, but a decrease in child problem behaviours known as 'meltdowns' and a willingness to share more with others were constantly recognised. Children too showed less separation anxiety when a dog was present.

Dogs were trained to touch the child's knee using 'target training' so that an impending repetitive head banging or a meltdown were defused by the dog's attentions. Studies of how reading skills in children improve were shown when the children can interact with a dog in the room, often reading aloud a selected book with a dog theme. In California, they had used a 'Paws for Tales' scheme in libraries encouraging the children to read aloud to the dog. Research programmes into the calming and motivational effects of dogs have been used in groups of six or seven students with low reading performance; the teacher brings their own dog into the class. Over a period of 12 weeks, the dog-assisted programme produces results to increase motivation: the best reader of the day is allowed to perform a trick with the dog and give a reward to the dog. Parents wrote of their satisfaction, including children's enjoyment of interacting with dogs and reading, and other benefits were the children's attachment to dogs, projection of their emotions onto dogs and the non-threatening and comfortable situation created by dogs in the classroom.

In England, reading skills may improve where a child has wanted to read stories to their dog, and hesitations whilst waiting to be corrected by a misread word are reduced when the dog is the only listener to the story. It was suggested that children should be asked to 'read to your dog' with the mother or carer just sitting beside the dog; this can improve a child's self-esteem and confidence in word recognition and speech. This is especially of use where a child faces language, learning or emotional challenges. The USA report stated that they had observed more interactions between the animal in eye contact, physical (touching) contact and speaking directly to the dog, which was always 'non-judgmental' about what was said. Attention spans were longer and hyperactive children were more ready to persevere in reading rather than getting up and running around; later the dog could join in the running about at the end of a session.

Exercise is important for general health, but the nature of a disability often limits exercise opportunities or restricts them to certain parts of the body. Authorities suggest that pet ownership in childhood may protect against obesity in all children. This in part could be due to the greater activity from playing and walking a dog, but there may be emotional benefits, and the example of the dog eating only regular meals acts as a control on food intake.

Children with special needs may have other dietary problems, but the dog can provide emotional support and encourage a child to eat in a similar style to the regular eating pattern of a companion dog. Research on overweight children at seven years, after controlling for gender, maternal education and social class, plus other previously identified risk factors for obesity in this group - birth weight, maternal smoking during pregnancy, parental obesity, TV watching, and sleep duration, obesity -was not associated with dog ownership. The role of the dog in reducing a tendency for the child to become overweight was quite minimal, apart from providing another source of comfort as a companion. Pet ownership alone would not protect against childhood obesity, which requires encouragement of a more active lifestyle and giving a benefit to emotional development.

Chapter 13

How dogs can help people with autistic spectrum disorders

One of the most innovative and remarkable developments was the use of assistance dogs to help people with autistic spectrum disorders (ASD). First reports came from North America of a new type of AAT using registered assistance dogs for children with specific needs associated with autism. Once the idea was introduced into Europe it rapidly gained popularity with parents as the specially trained dogs appeared to reduce the children's impulsiveness, self-harm, mood swings and social isolation especially when amongst other children in their age group. Having a dog was thought 'cool' and brought friendships through the dog's interactions: crawling around a child to calm him/her, alerting parents, responding to the child's verbal commands and reducing the risk of 'bolting' when outside the home were just some of the benefits parents would appreciate.

Using specifically-trained dogs to modify the social, language, and self-stimulatory behaviours specific to children with autism has been proved a success. The work in this new area was started in Canada in 1997 when a service dog was placed with a child with autism. National Service Dogs, a North American training organisation which had previously been training guide dogs for blind people, took up the challenge.

Chris Fowler spoke at the Assistance Dogs International Conference in 2008 about how he had first become involved in setting up the successful scheme to help ASD families. Out of 150 dogs then trained there were only four failures, marital 'split ups' being the commonest reason, he said.

A parent had approached Chris in Canada in 1996 to see if the training methods used in preparing guide dogs for the blind could be used to give his three-year-old son an assistance dog, even though there was no problem with the boy's vision. Later the Irish Guide Dog organisation was the first in Europe to follow the Canadian lead by using unsuited guide dogs to retrain for ASD children.

In the UK there had been reluctance by the Guide Dogs for the Blind Association to get involved with children; they had the capacity to widen their training skills but they continued with a rule not to issue a dog to anyone under 18 having a visual impairment. The age limit had been set many years previously. It was felt that a 'minor' could not legally be held responsible for the care or the welfare of a trained dog.

In this decade, the GDBA introduced Buddy Dogs in January 2012 for children who are partially sighted or blind. The ownership of the dog is transferred to the parents, but the dogs are not classified as assistance dogs so they do not have the access rights of guide dogs. Chris Fowler had been training guide dogs in Canada since 1994, before he prepared the first dog, a black Labrador, Shade, which was to be matched with an autistic child. The trainers in Ontario, Heather and Chris Fowler and Danielle Forbes, regularly used Labradors and Golden Retrievers in their work and they were employed at the first school in the world to provide this service of autism assistance.

Although Chris left the organisation to start with Autism Assistance Dog Guides in 2009, Danielle remains Executive Director of National Service Dogs with additional training courses set up for other neurobiological disorders such as PTSD for ex-service people.

Over the 18 years from 1996, NSD placed nearly 300 Certified Service Dogs across Canada for children and families living with autism. Animal Assistance Interventions (AAI) had been practised for many years among special needs persons. Dolphins were involved in the first animal interactions recorded with an autistic person, in 1984 Smith in the USA described using them to elicit communication from an autistic child. It was believed that the use of water and a non-threatening animal had created the beneficial changes observed in the child. There was a suspicion that dogs might react badly to abnormal human movements or behaviour, so the relationship was not further explored by marine-based organisations.

The more flexible approach in Canada allowed Chris Fowler to undertake training of a dog with a child. Fortunately the programme used was an almost immediate success, with an obvious response by the boy, and the decision was taken by National Service Dogs to train with more dogs for this specialised need of the many children with ASD. The training programme used in Canada was similar to a guide dog training programme, with socialising placement from puppies up to 12 months old within a foster family. There, basic obedience, socialisation within the family members and walking out of doors wearing a jacket helped the dog to get ready for the next stage, with advanced training from over 12 months lasting a further six to eight months at the centre's kennels. Obedience training, responding to the adult trainer, working the dog in busy town environments and supermarkets is aided by the positive reinforcement of reward giving when a task is done. Clicker training with positive reinforcement is used in the early stages, but this is phased out as reward giving has become sufficient incentive for the dog to complete the task.

The fully-trained service dogs in Canada were placed at 18 to 24 months of age after being matched to a child with autism, the parents or carer learning to work the dog during an initial training week at the NASD centre before bringing the dog home, when training continues with the child and other family members. The work Chris had done with children was described by Cliona O'Rourke, of the Irish Guide Dog organisation, who spoke at the Salzburg Conference in 2005: she had spent a year in Canada before coming back to Cork to start work with ASD dogs supported by Ken Brydon.

Another researcher group working with autism spectrum disorder in Italy, Pet Partners from the Scuola Cani Guida per Ciechi of Tuscany, found an improvement in the child's skills in behaviour, 'affective-relation communication' and improved motor skills that were most effective for the ASD group of children studied.

In recent years the recognition of the autism spectrum in young children has been seen to increase, most likely due to the better diagnosis of the condition. In fact, while many more cases may be seen in the total numbers now recorded, for reasons not yet fully understood the better medical analysis and diagnoses have revealed more autistic children who in the past were merely labelled as 'difficult' or at the worst 'mentally retarded'. This means that people with autism can be better cared for, especially where their condition is not seen as being in the unhelpful category of being 'naughty' or backward, but ASD is now seen as a specific developmental disorder.

There are three traits recognised which taken together constitute the spectrum condition: a problem with communication, difficulty in social integration and a pattern of repetitive behaviour. It is the second of these that dog pairing can help with most, but the first one is also improved as the child learns from the dog's communication methods (face, tail and other body responses). Even repetitive behaviour can be reduced by training the dog to react to the child's first signs, placing its head or paw on the child to redirect the child's attention. The child focuses onto the dog, with a concerned companion's interest in its behaviour.

Community involvement of the dog with a child brings benefits to everyone involved. The dog's jacket gives a message when seen out with any special needs person and it keeps everyone informed, helping the parents or carer to feel they are not just 'bad' or incompetent child raisers. It is an example of a low-level intervention that brings wide benefits.

Autism tendencies may be present in all humans to a lesser or greater degree, and ASD may be merely the extreme end of the normal state. Some people with Asperger's syndrome or mild autism are less affected when with others at work; others have such pronounced autistic behaviour that normal education and living independently are impossible.

Anything a dog can do at the formative stage of a child's development to allow integration with other children must have lifelong benefits, with considerable savings to the state in the continuing care needed for adults with the most severe autistic spectrum disorders. According to research on autism in Japan, dog owners experienced a rise of oxytocin hormone after playing with their dogs, or even after looking at them lovingly. The hormone produced warm calming feelings. Because it is a stress reducer, it dampens down an area in the brain that involves anxiety, which may account for many benefits of dog ownership for those in the autistic spectrum.

Animal Assistance Interventions and AAI in schools

The classroom can be a stressful and challenging environment for children with ASD as a major feature of this neurological disorder is an impairment in social interactions. A number of theorists and clinical practitioners have proposed that one attainable and viable addition to current classroom practices may be the implementation of AAI. It was hypothesized that AAI with dogs would increase positive social behaviours and decreases some problem behaviours in children with ASD. Attending a 'normal' school and being with other normally-developing peers potentially provides a unique outlet for children with ASD to socially integrate more fully with their classmates. Small pets such as guinea pigs have been brought into the classroom for two 30-minute sessions a week, so children aged between five and 12 years could work together grooming and caring for the animals. Placing one child with ASD to work with two classmates allowed for integration through improved social behaviours. They could watch the guinea pigs understand their physical needs and communicate by touch and voice with the animals, improving the social function of the children with ASD and relating in their peer groups with others.

Preliminary results suggest that AAI with dogs may provide a relatively simple and cost-effective means of helping educators and families to improve the social functioning of children with ASD. Dogs for the Disabled has worked with two schools where special educational needs children are beginning to see the benefit of a 'school dog' with an instructor regularly attending.

Registered Assistance Dogs with autistic children

As well as the 600 parents who have now attended the PAWS autism workshops organised through Dogs for the Disabled, there is a smaller number of autism assistance dogs trained at Dogs for the Disabled centres who can then meet the higher standard required by ADEu for access rights. The registered dogs then have the ability to be able to enter food stores or cafés and have the same rights as older people's qualified dogs.

Autism is a condition now known to have an inherited factor, but also with a strong early environment component in the way the condition develops. Defined as a neurological disorder that interferes with the normal development of the child, ASD could well be linked with early failure of bonding with adults and siblings. Such children were described by Enders-Siegers at the Utrecht Conference as 1) lacking verbal and non-verbal communicative skills, 2) also lacking imagination and not understanding humour very well and 3) sometimes displaying hyperactivity, running away or 'bolting' unexpectedly. More recently the absence of visual social skills has been recognised in ASD as to why children are unable to respond to normal cues for happiness or other emotions shown in the face or body of the persons closest to them, which in turn leads to a sense of isolation.

Animals are more straightforward in giving emotional cues, and the wagging tail is far more expressive than the slight changes in the human facial muscles that denote approval by adults or older children. Children find it easier to understand a dog's mouth when at their own eye level. The relaxed jaw of the dog, the position of the lips, a dangling tongue or body changes such as panting can all give readily-recognised messages to the child. The dog that has spent long enough in a play session with a child will just walk off quietly so the child recognises when 'enough is enough' to end a game without tears. By this understanding the relationship between dog and child is confidently strengthened and can produce a positive mood.

There are many moving stories of the effects of bringing a dog into the life of a person with a special need. I heard about Gunner and Lucy in November 2013 when I was in their home. Lucy's mother was not certain when I questioned her how she had first heard of the work of Dogs for the Disabled; a friend might have mentioned something about dogs helping children in this condition. Possibly it was soon after Lucy, aged two, had been confirmed as autistic by the paediatrician, the diagnosis being made within 20 minutes of her first appointment at the clinic.

After this confirmation of the parents' own observations on their non-verbal daughter, an internet search led the family to Dogs for the Disabled's web site and an application was made in late 2012. After the mother had attended an information day at the Banbury centre with others to hear about 'Autism Dogs', quite soon afterwards she was pleased to be selected for a dog. Instructor Kelly brought along Gunner, a black Labrador, to the house so she could welcome him, and she later came to love him when he moved into her home.

The next step in acquiring an assistance dog was for Lucy's mother to spend a week in residence at the Frances Hay Centre. With several other mothers of autistic children, she was taught to understand what her dog needs would be: toilet training, regular meals and of course, exercise. This meant walking on the lead at the required pace for a small child and observing how Gunner had been trained to stand still as soon as any person attached to his harness attempted to run off or 'bolt'. After successfully completing all the tasks, she was allowed to take Gunner home with her for the weekend and next Gunner moved into the household permanently. Qualification walks from the home formed part of the assessment of the partnership with the dog. Once qualified, access to food shops, stores and to other public places was possible for Gunner, as he was then a registered assistance dog.

The first meeting of little Lucy with Gunner was in her own home and it was one of cautious apprehension, her mother told me. Later on she would respond to the antics of the dog, which was still young, when playing out in the garden. Lucy showed this by excited laughter at the freedom of activity that Gunner enjoyed when off the lead.

Lucy's older sister helped with this new introduction to the family; later on she would take Gunner into her bedroom at night to read him stories which he listened to, waiting for the reward in the form of a food treat! This was especially of value whilst Lucy's mother had the sometimes difficult task of getting her ready for bed and off to sleep in the evening.

From the time Gunner arrived in May 2013, the relationship between dog and child developed quite slowly. Walks were taken with Gunner and the two children. Lucy was attached by a waistband to Gunner's harness, which she held by an attached handle. No longer was there the fear that Lucy would shoot off into the main road outside the home. Walks previously had been quite frequent when the pushchair was used, but once Lucy grew bigger, she wanted to walk on her own. It was always a concern that she might run off if she was not firmly held, and she got anxious when in new unfamiliar places, but Gunner was helping to overcome these problems too.

At the age of three Lucy started attending nursery school two half days a week. Here an unexpected function of Gunner was that other children and their parents could see Lucy was 'special' as she had a dog, wearing a jacket, to meet her after school. Lucy started full-time school in September 2014 and settled in well, her mother told me. She had started to use a few recognisable words now and was progressing socially too, playing more with her sister and peers. Lucy learnt how to brush Gunner and play 'high fives' paw raising with him; Gunner enjoys ball games and Lucy is generally more aware of things going on around her. Perhaps one day Gunner will be able to attend during some lessons to give Lucy even more confidence.

Other benefits of having a trained assistance dog in the home affected the whole family. Excursions became easier, such as a visit to McDonalds' where Lucy sat quietly until the end of the meal because Gunner was tucked in beside her lying under the table. Family holidays at the seaside were less difficult when the now familiar Gunner was travelling with Lucy. She could reassure herself by touching Gunner's head or body as she walked past and he did not object; speech is still awaited, but it is hoped that one day Lucy will talk to her dog, perhaps when out on a walk. Some games, such as ball throwing and retrieval, are fairly easy to develop to help in the attachment process, but time is necessary to allow a young child to progress in the same way as older children with an assistance dog. Regular short walks, such as the one down to the postbox, form part of the daily routine. As Lucy gets older, longer walks are planned and more excursions into the town will follow.

Another autism dog I met in the home was Nala, working with Sam. Sam's mother Julie told me how the dog fitted into their rather crowded house, more so since the return of an older son who had started a postgraduate university course. Julie told me in December 2013 that Sam is a non-verbal 'high functioning' ASD boy, attending a special school some 20 miles from his home (travelling from Kenilworth to Stratford daily). He is now 11 years old and very good at mathematics, but with physical problems affecting his walking. There had previously been two pet dogs in the family, but none since they had moved houses. They were now living in the same area as where Frances Hay started assistance dogs in 1988.

Sam's mother found out about guide dogs working with the blind only when they moved into the area, but later she conducted internet searches and found the organisation in Banbury that trained ASD dogs. The family had lived in the Kenilworth area for 15 years, having come from Lancashire, so they knew nothing about how Dogs For the Disabled had started with its first assistance dog in that part of Warwickshire in 1988.

Julie learnt more about the organisation when she went to an invitation day at the Banbury kennels in October 2011, four months after her first enquiries. She liked what she heard from other parents there and filled in the necessary application forms. Within a few months she had a visit to her home from one of the instructors who brought along with her a dog. Julie later said she had first heard about dogs working with autistic children through the speech therapist at the primary school: that was in May 2011, when the therapist said she too had only just learnt about them. Julie read everything possible about assistance dogs before making the application to Dogs for the Disabled. When she went to one of the craft fairs held at the Banbury training centre and kennels, she could talk to the mother of a child who had received an ASD dog, which convinced her that she had made the right decision in making an application.

In May 2012 Julie heard her application had been successful, because of her previous experience with dogs and the fact that she was 'not fussy about the colour of the dog'. She thought she had not had to wait as long as other applicants.

Sam had met Nala at a matching visit to the home, which had gone well: Sam was lying on the floor, Nala was wagging her tail in his face and he was laughing from this first contact. Being non-verbal, Sam gave his 'thumbs up' sign, the way he showed his approval of the dog coming to the home. Julie next went to Banbury to stay at the centre for the week of residential training. There she learnt what the dog required and how it had been trained, so that she could make the best use of it when she took Nala home on the Friday evening. They found Sam was much calmer after the dog came, and being able to go out as a family to a restaurant to eat a meal was the first major change in family life. Sam had previously needed tube feeding due to his multiple disabilities; he would now eat, but then quickly got bored and restless. Once when on holiday before the dog came, there was an incident where Sam had run out of the restaurant as soon as the meal came to the table and went straight into the main road before he could be stopped. With Nala in a restaurant Sam would sit quietly with the rest of the family as he knew she was waiting under the table as the others finished their food.

Other parents too had found holidays were difficult and a time of unpredictable actions which did not encourage relaxation. The dog's harness, which made a connection between parent and dog and from dog to child, made activity more predictable. When Sam was at home, going out for walks was no longer an ordeal with Nala present. When away from the house his mother said he had a huge smile on his face, and Sam walked quicker, striding away when he was with Nala. Previously he had walked slowly and at one time he had worn leg callipers, but his mother said 'with Nala in the harness he thinks he is in charge and seems proud of the dog'. School writings too confirmed his appreciation: statements like 'I love my dog' and 'Nala is my dog' showed his expression of contentment.

At school and in the home, computers and mathematics were Sam's strong interest. Previously his fascination with numbers would show on walks where he would reach out to see any car number plates, even going out into the road to get closer. The longer the numbers on the plate the better, so older cars were of greater interest than the newer ones. Now with the waistband connection to Nala, this was no longer a problem. Julie said there had been no negative aspects, and the whole family was more relaxed.

Sam's 17-year-old brother also lived at home and the eldest boy was studying for an International Technology Management Masters at university, so the house became quite full at times. 'Everyone in the family just adores Nala, she never barks at anyone', he said.

Nala sees her puppy socialiser, Claire, from time to time, and she is also delighted to see how well Nala has fitted into her new family home life. There are other stories about the benefits of having a dog and in the last chapter we will hear about Claude in a daily account written by a parent of an ASD boy. Twenty-five years ago autism was still regarded as a rare and obscure disorder, often put together with 'mentally handicapped' in diagnosis and effective treatment was rarely provided; long-term institutional care was have been society's response, rather than treatment. Residential schools aimed to minimise ASD triggers, but one parent wrote: 'I see my 17-year-old son hitting himself viciously on the head and screaming when he can't cope with a noise that upsets him. Sometimes the outbursts are directed at the carer. His language ability was of an 18-month-old and he had the emotional stability of a three-year-old. When he is home on visits his sisters are scared when he comes and make excuses not to be in'.

Fortunately, autism is now recognised widely. It has become a common assessment, with one in a hundred children in the western world affected. High-functioning autism has often been associated with unreasonable or unexplained human behaviours and linked to talent creativity and mathematical feats. Some are just people who are different from the norm, such as Alan Turing, who has been reassessed for his genius as a mathematician and code breaker.

Although there have been considerable advances in the study of genetics and disease tendencies, neuroscience still has to make headway in elucidating the mediating links or in suggesting the best therapeutic interventions. The increased awareness and diagnosis of autism appears to be largely a cultural trend towards redefining human differences, recognising a disorder. Assistance dogs have helped to alter the perception of ASD. Parents are no longer made to feel guilty or blamed for making their children autistic through their aloofness and frigid personality, as they were at one time in the post-war decade.

There is currently much research into the reasons for and the factors affecting a person's development in the autistic spectrum. There was a suggestion recently that higher levels of testosterone in the prenatal period were associated with autistic behaviour patterns; the left side of the forebrain is involved in language and the right forebrain deals with emotional information. Where the hind part of the brain processes information, if some of the pathways were missing that connect to the two sides of the forebrain, then signs may develop of

ASD. An inherited factor may also be involved in neurological pathways not developing fully but more research is required into the condition.

Those in the autistic spectrum may fail to see the body language of others around them. The way people with ASD see and process body language could prevent them from gauging the feelings of others, adding to their difficulties with social interaction. In a study by Durham University, when adults with ASD watched short video clips of body movements without facial expressions or sounds, they found it hard to identify emotions such as anger or happiness. Those who struggled most with this task also performed poorly at detecting the direction in which a group of dots moved on a screen, indicating a problem with visual processing.

Mark Haddon's book *The Curious Incident of the Dog in the Nighttime* and the film *Rain Man* improved public recognition of the peculiar and until then almost unknown behaviours that made up the autistic life of many. A correspondent to a national newspaper over five years ago commented: 'The increased diagnosis of the condition has led people to believe that there was an epidemic in the prevalence of autism and fears were attributed to introduced poisons and vaccines, to name two. The religious element of being possessed by the Devil had long since vanished although for a long time in the 20th century a nervous twitch was named 'St Vitus' Dance' as if there had been a demonic possession of the child. Desperate parents have fallen in to using miracle 'cures' and institutional therapies with the expectation of driving out some inner force or detoxification of the brain. 'Normalising' autism may reduce the stigma but at the risk of trivialisation the problem for those with more severe autistic spectrum disorder manifestations. And also increasing the extreme aloneness that that results from social impairment of autism even in high functioning adults'.

Another *Times* writer, writing at the same time over five years, ago added 'My son's ASD is an almost invisible condition for the majority of those who come across him. He simply cannot understand the rules of social interaction, resulting in 'inappropriate' behaviour that can cause an insensitive response from even those close acquaintances. It is hard to express the hurt and damage to self-esteem inflicted by those who make implied or explicit criticism of our parenting skills'.

There are huge challenges from ASD and anything that can help the public to appreciate that a child who is behaving 'badly' might not just be a spoiled brat could avoid demoralising interventions and lead to greater community and family support. Self-stimulatory behaviours such as head banging, a lack of social reciprocity and language deficits could be alarming. Bystanders would give inappropriate responses and imply that it was a lack of parental skill that was at fault. Tantrums on the supermarket floor were difficult to explain to other shoppers, but if the public were made aware of the condition by the presence of a dog with an assistance dog jacket, it would help the watchers of an event to appreciate that the child was not a spoilt kid but one who needed an assistance dog's presence to get along with life. Very often the parents or carers express great relief that the trained dog has led to greater community involvement and wider family support.

The responses made by ASD children in the presence of a dog may often be inconclusive, but usually benefits are seen in the family where a dog is introduced. The two letters were written before assistance dogs were becoming known to help in the conditions described, and now in mid-2015 there has been a considerable improvement in public awareness of the condition. Although autism came to the fore with increased diagnoses made since 1900, there is some evidence that it was a disease in antiquity, influencing art and artefacts in the ice age in Europe. Autism may have helped to bring in new skills into human society when living conditions for a person with ASD would have been less complicated in a simpler world.

AAII

Animal Assistance Intervention International is a non-profit organisation that provides greater awareness of dogs and other animals being used in treatments. Founded in 2013, it attempts to coordinate people involved with therapies and to maintain professional standards.

The different forms of assistance that dogs give often confuse the public when the abbreviations AAT, AAI and AAA are used indiscriminately. The Society for Companion Animal Studies (SCAS) made clear with definitions the different forms of these activities. AAI, or Animal-Assisted Interventions, are any intervention that intentionally includes or incorporates animals as part of a therapeutic or ameliorative process, as was described by Kruger and Serpell in 2006. The term AAI includes 'animal-assisted activities' (AAA) and 'animal-assisted therapy' (AAT). Many people working in the field adopted the Delta Society (now Pet Partners) definitions to differentiate between these two approaches:

AAA - Animal-assisted activities: these provide opportunities for motivational, educational, recreational and/or therapeutic benefits to enhance quality of life. AAAs are delivered in a variety of environments by paraprofessionals and/or volunteers in association with animals that meet specific criteria. Interactions are spontaneous and there is no requirement to document or evaluate. There is no goal or end point set by the therapist.

AAT - Animal-assisted therapy: a goal-directed intervention in which an animal that meets specific criteria is an integral part of the treatment process. AAT is directed and/or delivered by a health/human service professional with specialised expertise and within the scope of practice of his/her profession. Outcomes are documented, measured and evaluated.

AAT has been developed worldwide with good results. In the USA 14 clinical trials on the effects of AAT on children affected with ASD were analysed, and 30 different outcome variables showed statistically that there were significant improvements in 27 of the 30 measured. The publication suggested that the dog trained to assist a person with autism might give to the person the same support services as a dog that was specially trained for those who were blind or deaf. They stated that an assistance dog alerts the partner to distracting repetitive movements common among those with autism, allowing the person to stop the movement (eg, hand flapping, head nodding). A person with autism may have problems with sensory input and need a dog to interpret the actions of others and events around the person. The approach adopted for a programme using an assistance dog will depend on whether it is goal-directed or spontaneous, delivered by a trained health care professional (eg a counsellor, occupational therapist) or a volunteer and if it is documented, evaluated and measured. The Behavioural Inventory (PDDBI) used as the baseline in research and later follow-ups measures the child's level of functioning but it may need to be continued for years. Research on autism and other brain disorders continues in many countries, but the place of assistance dogs seems firmly established.

Chapter 14

PAWS – helping more children with special needs

Dogs for the Disabled had 25 years' experience of putting into practice the idea of dogs as helpers in disability, as well as having collected considerable knowledge on dog training in special situations. The staff had developed their skills in interviewing and assessing those most suited to have a trained assistance dog and working out how to provide the best support. With the 2004 success of the first two dogs trained specifically for children, there were new opportunities to make dogs available to more families who had one, or sometimes more, children with some form of disability. One trainer could provide dogs for an instructor to produce about eight dogs a year for the children's assistance dog team project. There were many enquiries flooding in from those who had read magazine articles or seen features on TV about special needs children who had dogs with them at home.

The trustees of Dogs for the Disabled held a special one-day meeting to look at how assistant dog services could be expanded to meet this new demand. There had been renewed media interest, and more donations came in as the appeal of children and dogs brought together made for greater success in fundraising. An information service was suggested where dog-related questions were answered, where to find help and how to choose a dog, and answers could be obtained via the internet or over the phone. This would encourage thousands of families to train their own dog to help a member of the family with autistic spectrum disorder. As a low-cost way of spreading the greater use of assistance dogs, it had many attractions; it only needed funding for one person, possibly someone with a disability, who could be employed to operate the enquiry and information service.

Peter Gorbing, with his many contacts, was able to interest a philanthropist living in Australia who would be prepared to finance a better scheme. Mel Gottlieb, through a trust fund called Response Systems International, was able to set up finance for an innovative scheme for dog training, to be known as Parents Autism Workshops & Support (PAWS). Funding for a three-year project would allow for meetings of parents in groups, to tell them how they could help themselves to have trained dogs and ensure continuing support was available at the end of the trial period.

Peter told the press: 'There are hundreds of families we could help', referring to the successes of launching PAWS. It was considered that three all-day meetings spaced out at intervals would give sufficient time to impart the necessary information. Live dogs would be used for demonstrations and instruction given on how parents could match dogs to individual ASD children's requirements. Over the first three years, 600 families were able to benefit through the one individual's generosity.

PAWS proved an immediate success in 2010; two experienced dog trainers were engaged and they travelled to various centres in England and Wales. Carers and parents who applied were directed to attend one of the day-long classes that were being arranged across the country to demonstrate how a dog could be prepared to help an autistic child. Some of those coming to the meetings already had a dog and wanted to know how to interact better with a child and a dog. Others who had recently heard about PAWS wanted to know the right sort of puppy to buy or acquire from a rescue kennels. The instructors' talks gave information on how to prepare the dog with basic training, and how to socialise the young dog so it would be relaxed in the home; the next stage was building a up a solid relationship with members of the family, especially giving support to the child with ASD.

Spread over months, the one-day workshops were held at each location, spaced out, so they would be sufficient to start parents or carers in the best way possible for the effective use of dogs in the home. These courses led to many more families being able to use dogs in a more targeted way than if they had just been left on a waiting list of one or two other charities providing autism assistance dogs. The meetings were structured to give opportunities for parents to discuss issues of responsible dog ownership, dog training and working with a family dog to support behaviour modification in the child. The results of PAWS classes were described favourably by one commentator: 'We conclude that pet contact improves basal social skills in children, repetitive behaviours such as head nodding could be interrupted when the dog distracted the child and a dog would increase confidence when away from the home'.

Parents' expectations of what dogs might do were deliberately kept low; an earlier experience in 2006 had been with a mother whose son had been diagnosed with ASD. She came to Banbury for a week's residential training with the dog but her expected lifestyle improvement was not met by what a dog might do in the home: the dog was withdrawn from use after quite a short time. Fortunately there was the opportunity to issue the same dog later to another family with an ASD boy and this time it was a successful partnership.

One of the first successes was with William with his mother Helen, who became a very effective partnership working with the black

Labrador Percy. The boy's new confidence when walking out with the dog was used in a promotional video for Dogs for the Disabled's work, and the use of the waist belt from the boy to the dog and the longer lead from the adult carer to the dog were clearly shown in the film. William and Percy were finalists in the Friends for Life Award at Crufts and the publicity meant the charity was again receiving more enquiries about getting a ready-trained dog which led to the launching of the PAWS scheme.

At this time, 42% of the applications for assistance dogs made to Dogs for the Disabled were coming in from the parents of ASD children. The demand could only be met if the parents and carers were introduced to PAWS, as a quicker method of training an assisting dog for an ASD offspring. The charity benefited financially too from publicity from working with children, and received £88,000 in new donations after it launched its autism dogs programme, which enabled the training of eight additional assistance dogs.

The PAWS workshops were set up at 15 centres in England and enquirers were directed to the place nearest to their home. The parent(s) or carers were invited to the first of three one-day instruction sessions. The Dogs Trust and some dog clubs were able to offer training hall space for each class organised. It was decided not to ask the children to attend nor for people to bring their own pet dogs along, since these would be distractions for those coming to learn from the dog trainers. Kate Bristow, one of the first PAWS workshop leaders, explained: 'PAWS is different from other animal-assisted interaction projects that were tried before because it is aimed to bring out the best in the family relationship with a pet dog'. The PAWS scheme was also taken up in Australia and the Netherlands and more recently schemes have started in Belgium and in Spain.

When members of a family with an autistic child attend a PAWS meeting in their region, they were asked to come with a companion but neither a child nor a dog. The two instructors first showed what a demonstration dog could do and games with the dogs were encouraged. Advice on choosing a suitable dog, often with the help of rescue centre kennels, integrating it into the whole family and task training were all covered over the three days. One adult in the household was given ultimate responsibility for the care and the welfare of the dog. Clicker training was shown, a new method for many pet owners, and positive reward-based dog training was encouraged.

It was important to have a settling-in period and friends and visitors were discouraged in the early days to help make the change of home as stress-free for the dog as possible. It had to be explained that the dogs did not have the full access rights of qualified assistance dogs, but often it was enough to say 'it's been trained like an assistance dog' for the dog in a jacket to be made welcome in cafés or other public places. Visits to food shops and supermarkets were not permitted as the dogs had not undergone the rigorous health checks of all the other assistance dogs trained by AD (UK) member organisations, nor did they get the six-monthly aftercare visits made to registered assistance dogs.

The experience of PAWS for one mother and her two children Jude and Gabe was described in her account, written five years ago. The blog gives a vivid description of what a difference a dog could make in a difficult home situation. She wrote at the time:

'This is a long-overdue post about Claude, our beautiful, biddable, chilled but chipper, lifesaver of a Labrador. I've meant to write about him for a good two years - I've stood up in front of roomfuls of real-live grown up people twice now to talk about him for fundraisers for Dogs for the Disabled (more on that later) but somehow words have evaded me here up till now. Claude is now a fully-grown dog of two.

He's gorgeous; he's a family therapist, chief comforter, arbitrator, speech therapist, marriage guidance counsellor, jester, personal trainer and all round good egg. The phrase 'man's best friend' doesn't come from nowhere. He is man, woman and boys' best friend around here (actually cat's as well - he and our feisty feline, Sass, are inseparable). He is my constant companion and rock - happy to share my joys and put up with any teary down days. He's always delighted to see any one of us and even half an hour's absence merits a full hopping, wagging, toothy-grinning greeting from Claude. He considers it his duty to see J onto the school bus in the mornings and to sit waiting by the gate for him - rain or shine - when he returns. He hops into bed with G for his morning cuddles while I get J up and ready. He is gentle and patient and has 'turned' many a dog-phobic child into one who clamours for his very own Claude!

'It all started when we were wading about in the seeming quagmire of J's new diagnosis. As an antidote to the reams of medical jargon, 'cures' and therapies that I'd been trailing through, I read a book called 'A Friend Like Henry' that my sister had sent me. It is the story of a family wrestling with their son's fairly severe autism whose lives were turned around by getting a dog. This lovely (and true) story prompted the next flurry of Googling and researching and we came across 'Autism Assistance Dogs'. These dogs are incredible - trained to keep the kids safe, break tantrums and to be friends to kids with autism - but, sadly, extremely few and far between in this country - only 2 organisations are currently training these remarkable creatures (Dogs for the Disabled being one) and the waiting lists are enormous. Along with the fact that Dave and I are hideously impatient people, we also decided that a dog to specifically help J would only serve to tip the precarious balance of our family even further at that point. What we really wanted was something to take the prime focus of our lives off J's autism and to help us to be us again - G needed a canine friend just as much as J and, actually, so did we!

'More Googling led to the discovery that not all breeders are happy to hand over a puppy to a family containing a child with autism – 'that's mental illness isn't it - sorry love, couldn't do that to a dog'! However, we'd learnt early on in J's life that our gut feelings tend to be worth sticking with, and having decided that only a Black Labrador would do, I persisted until we found the beautiful Poppy and her pups, residing in palatial splendour on the Putney banks of the River Thames. Poppy's owner couldn't have been more helpful and invited us to bring G and J over to hang out with the puppies. After all, J had never even so much as glanced at a dog so we had no idea whether he'd even like creatures of a canine persuasion. While G and I melted into fits of cooing over Claude and his plump, wagging siblings, J took no interest whatsoever and wandered off down the garden. This complete lack of interest was by no means reciprocated by Poppy who had volunteered herself as J's guardian for the entire duration of our visit. She was never more than a whisker away from him for the hour that we were there. When J sat down, Poppy sat down. When J ran, Poppy ran. Now and again J would place a hand on her head, without looking at her. There was some kind of magic going on here and, being scientific types (!), that was good enough for me and Dave.

'A few weeks, many visual schedules and 'social stories' later, along with J's now obsessive viewing of the video clips we'd made of the puppies, we collected a 12-week-old Claude. And that was the first day that J ever spoke to anyone directly. 'Hello Claude. You are a dog' - full (and I mean full) eye contact, along with blushes of delight as he bustled around finding toys for our new family member and occasionally rushed off to his letter bricks to spell out his new best friend's name. It didn't take long for the blanket of love that Claude inspired to envelop us and pretty much everyone who met him.

'Those first few months were by no means plain sailing - it was a lot of fun but tougher lessons were also learnt - cause/effect being one of them when J discovered that if you pull Claude's ears/tail then he squeaks pleasingly. Up to this point, J hadn't associated the pain that he felt when he was hurt in any way with pain that others felt. In autism there is a classic lack of empathy so if J yanked out a handful of my hair and I screamed or if the puppy had his tail pulled and squeaked, J didn't understand that the pain we felt was the same sensation as the pain he felt when he bashed his head/knee etc. I totally drew the line at Claude being hurt so made a very clear rule and a rather fine 'social story' about why we don't hurt others and spent several weeks never more than a foot away from J when he was near Claude to prevent any repeat offences - it was knackering but it worked.

'The other benefits and lessons are too many and varied to go into in too much detail (that dog deserves a book really) but in short: Claude's toilet training gave J's toilet training the impetus it had hitherto lacked - J finally realised that neither he nor the dog would be praised for peeing in a glorious arc across the living room! He also discovered that pee comes from within and is not just a disconnected wet feeling hitting your feet - this after much scrutiny of Claude's 'demonstrations'! Both boys basked in the loyalty that Claude provided - their squeals of mirth and merriment would bring Claude running to join in the fun, just as their tears and traumas would bring a wagging Claude to rescue them from their woes.

'When out and about with a roly-poly puppy, it is impossible to avoid PEOPLE. The world loves a puppy, and however much J would like those people to keep their puppy stroking, cooing gooeyness to themselves, the lure of those brown eyes and a wagging tail is too strong for these people. J had to get used to the fact that when we were out with Claude, people would come and talk to us. It took quite some time for him to become accustomed to this 'intrusion' but eventually he began to tolerate it.

'Children with autism can be tenacious and obsessive. Small puppies can be tenacious and obsessive. Give them a tug of war toy and they'll amuse each other for at least an hour. Having a small defenceless puppy in the family finally stopped every conversation that me and Dave had being about autism and kids - we'd been floundering about, trying to come to terms with J's autism and it was somewhat engulfing us. But somehow, by adding in the rhythm of having to walk, feed and water the dog, we managed to break the loop we'd got stuck in. Suffice to say that we were all pretty chuffed with Claude. He excelled at his training classes, was easy and fun to take out for walks and was happy to be mobbed at the school gates by his very own fan club of kids.

'At that point Dogs for the Disabled contacted us, inviting us onto the pilot scheme for a course they were setting up, not for autism assistance dogs, but for their PAWS workshops. There was a general guide to getting the right dog (OK so we'd done this bit and realised we'd been pretty lucky with Claude - not all dogs would be fit for the task); and then, more interestingly to me, a large chunk of the workshops was working with D for D's dogs and being shown how to maximise the relationship between a child with autism and a pet dog. I loved these workshops - the Dogs for the Disabled people really know their stuff and clearly all adore their work. They have a huge enthusiasm for what they do and their methods of training the dogs are fascinating. Using a clicker (little metal thing that makes a clicky sound which indicates that the dog is doing it right, precipitating a tasty reward) - breaking the tasks into tiny, achievable segments and allowing the dogs to work out for themselves what it is that you want them to do, rewarding them grandly at each stage. It is a very gentle way of training, and the dogs LOVE it. I thought it would take ages for Claude to pick up all this training but within half an hour of using these methods with him at home, he was getting the hang of it nicely. By the end of the first month of using these methods, Claude could do the following task: touch his nose to J, when he was having a meltdown; no mean feat with all the yelling and flailing around that goes with this. The point is not for Claude to make like Nanny McPhee and stop the tantrum, but rather for this little soft nudge to give a nanosecond of a pause in J's distress, allowing me to get in and calm him down. Claude was happy to walk on a double lead, with J holding onto one handle and me holding the other - a total revelation for me to have all the family going in the same direction at the same time!

'Claude helped in many situations. Modelling any new or 'offensive' items of clothing that J is refusing to wear (a school tie being a good example); causing much amusement all round and the eventual acceptance of the clothes by J. Demonstrating with gusto how to sample a new, unfamiliar food type and Claude could play the keyboard with his nose! OK, so not strictly what PAWS classes had advised, but me and G had a high old time teaching him this and he was mighty proud of his musical prowess!

'The simplest trip out can be fraught with danger. Being a superhero, J is not a keen hand holder and has a slippery superpower of being able to almost dislocate his shoulders/wrists in a bid to escape, if grabbed. He doesn't like to walk at the same pace as the rest of us and normally trails about 20 yards behind, favouring the outermost kerb stones to hop along. As 'Danger Boy' he has been known to skip, without warning, into oncoming traffic and likes to balance on brick walls and bollards.

'With or without specialist training, Claude would always have been an exceptional dog. The PAWS training showed us how to get the most out of the relationship between a child with autism and a hound, and that is the point. It is a relationship, an exceedingly strong one - not always noticeable to the naked eye but a very unconditional one. Most of us have so many relationships - with family, friends,

241

teachers, colleagues, people on the street, etc, etc - that we can hardly count them. J's 'tribe' is much smaller than most and will probably remain so for the rest of his life. Give him some pens and paper or a child to play with and he'd go for the first option every time. This is who he is and, although what he lacks in natural understanding of human relationships, he will be able to learn by rote in the future, I believe that he will always be happiest with just a few trusted tribe-members and Claude is certainly one of the chosen few. That dog is truly part of our family and, looking at him - fast asleep, legs in the air, jowls dream-eating something delicious, the boy snuggled into his neck, I couldn't imagine any more effective 'cure' for our family.'

More recently Kristina wrote about Claude again, now six and a half years old and still performing well as an autism assistance dog.

'Claude is still a much-loved and vital member of our family. Our boys are growing up and some of the old challenges have waned and been replaced by new challenges (Gabe is 13 years old and a fully-fledged teenager). Jude is nearly 10 and holds onto to Claude's lead when we are out and about – we don't use the double lead any more because I can 100% trust Claude to stop at crossings and not chase after anything tempting (we have kept up the level of training over the years). When Jude is holding the lead, Claude seems to know instinctively that he is on duty and acts accordingly. Similarly, when Jude is holding the lead, it 'grounds' him and reminds him that he has to walk calmly. Claude also continues to be there to mop up any tears on bad days – from both boys. His wagging, doe-eyed presence helps to remind both boys that somebody loves them and I genuinely believe that this has taught them a bit of empathy.

'The routines of dog ownership fit our life perfectly – Claude needs walking and feeding at specific times and this gels our days together too. He and I walk miles daily and I think we both see this as our 'time off'! Claude often reminds me of the Rudyard Kipling poem 'If' – he is a calm and non-judgmental presence in our lives. Dogs like Claude are most certainly not a 'cure' for autism but they are soothing, loving, wagging balm for families who are struggling through 'bad days' (despite the mud and dog hairs that have become part of the fabric of our house). We feel so grateful to have him and to have discovered from the PAWS workshops, the extent of how much difference dogs can make to some children's lives.'

PAWS and skilled companion teams

Many hundreds of others were able to take advantage of the PAWS training. Although they were not able to get the full access rights of a registered assistance dog, it enabled 'the team' of the carer and the ASD child to gain recognition and take advantage of a new increased awareness of other forms of disability other than those in wheelchairs. It had been necessary to get special written consent from the Charity Commission, in September 2006, to enable this development with PAWS to take place. A resolution at the General Meeting of Dogs for Disabled was also required to alter the constitution by adding in the words: 'by provision of practical and information-based services to support disabled people, who have, or wish to have, a dog'. It was something Frances Hay would not have thought possible but it was entirely in keeping with her wish to have dogs helping disabled and disadvantaged children as well as adults.

Some of the things that benefit the PAWS teams were found by experience: dogs would be the recipients' chance to share private thoughts, such as when dealing with emotional issues, a non-judgmental friend to watch but not try to correct. The opportunity for observing the dog's willingness to be toilet trained and develop eating at the regular family feeding times. Dogs wishing to be active when not sleeping, they would encourage physical activity with all the health benefits associated with exercise, and the dog would also entice other children to join in with games and play. The dog would show its loyalty to the ASD child but other children could come round to share in some of the companionship a dog can offer, especially if the other children had no pets in their own home.

Children developed increased confidence and improved self-esteem, as the dog would take the child as he or she was and not make comparisons with other children in the same age group or school class. As we found in the early days by wheelchair users, people come to talk as the dog is the 'ice breaker', overcoming the embarrassment of those first meeting disability in others. Dogs became important to bring 'social inclusion' rather than creating barriers that lead to exclusions. Other benefits found were in reducing stress levels, the immune system functions better improving general health, while trying out new foods in the way the dog does helped to improve self-imposed dietary restrictions. The dog's loyalty and devotion improves the child's attention span, visiting clinics was made easier when a dog was present and it helped with pain relief for some procedures.

A dog can encourage skills and a sense of sharing: practical problem solving was encouraged. The child can develop strategies getting the most out of the dogs' presence and can help the child to come to terms with some of the restrictions of disability. Parents and carers too found the dog being in the home had a good influence and would help to defuse tense moments in the day. It was a very powerful endorsement of the positive and unique impact dogs can have on human lives. Frances Hay could never have dreamed that within a few decades of the start of her work, Assistance Dogs for Disabled People would be used so extensively and in so many new situations.

From October 15 2015, Dogs for the Disabled will be known as Dogs for Good, with the same registered charity number 1092960.

Index of Names

S

T

V

W

SUBJECT INDEX

23948479R00158

Printed in Great Britain
by Amazon